Diagnosis of Neurogenetic Disorders

Diagnosis of Neurogenetic Disorders: Contribution of Next Generation Sequencing and Deep Phenotyping

Special Issue Editor
Alisdair McNeill

MDPI • Basel • Beijing • Wuhan • Barcelona • Belgrade

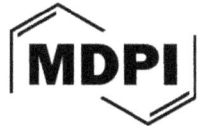

Special Issue Editor
Alisdair McNeill
University of Sheffield
UK

Editorial Office
MDPI
St. Alban-Anlage 66
4052 Basel, Switzerland

This is a reprint of articles from the Special Issue published online in the open access journal *Brain Sciences* (ISSN 2076-3425) from 2018 to 2019 (available at: https://www.mdpi.com/journal/brainsci/special_issues/diagnosis_neurogenetic_disorders).

For citation purposes, cite each article independently as indicated on the article page online and as indicated below:

LastName, A.A.; LastName, B.B.; LastName, C.C. Article Title. *Journal Name* **Year**, *Article Number*, Page Range.

ISBN 978-3-03921-610-9 (Pbk)
ISBN 978-3-03921-611-6 (PDF)

© 2019 by the authors. Articles in this book are Open Access and distributed under the Creative Commons Attribution (CC BY) license, which allows users to download, copy and build upon published articles, as long as the author and publisher are properly credited, which ensures maximum dissemination and a wider impact of our publications.

The book as a whole is distributed by MDPI under the terms and conditions of the Creative Commons license CC BY-NC-ND.

Contents

About the Special Issue Editor vii

Alisdair McNeill
Editorial for *Brain Sciences* Special Issue: "Diagnosis of Neurogenetic Disorders: Contribution of Next-Generation Sequencing and Deep Phenotyping"
Reprinted from: *Brain Sci.* **2019**, *9*, 72, doi:10.3390/brainsci9030072 1

Jennifer F. Gardner, Thomas D. Cushion, Georgios Niotakis, Heather E. Olson, P. Ellen Grant, Richard H. Scott, Neil Stoodley, Julie S. Cohen, Sakkubai Naidu, Tania Attie-Bitach, Maryse Bonnières, Lucile Boutaud, Férechté Encha-Razavi, Sheila M. Palmer-Smith, Hood Mugalaasi, Jonathan G. L. Mullins, Daniela T. Pilz and Andrew E. Fry
Clinical and Functional Characterization of the Recurrent TUBA1A p.(Arg2His) Mutation
Reprinted from: *Brain Sci.* **2018**, *8*, 145, doi:10.3390/brainsci8080145 3

Christopher Buckley, Lisa Alcock, Ríona McArdle, Rana Zia Ur Rehman, Silvia Del Din, Claudia Mazzà, Alison J. Yarnall and Lynn Rochester
The Role of Movement Analysis in Diagnosing and Monitoring Neurodegenerative Conditions: Insights from Gait and Postural Control
Reprinted from: *Brain Sci.* **2019**, *9*, 34, doi:10.3390/brainsci9020034 15

Emilia M. Gatto, Gustavo Da Prat, Jose Luis Etcheverry, Guillermo Drelichman and Martin Cesarini
Parkinsonisms and Glucocerebrosidase Deficiency: A Comprehensive Review for Molecular and Cellular Mechanism of Glucocerebrosidase Deficiency
Reprinted from: *Brain Sci.* **2019**, *9*, 30, doi:10.3390/brainsci9020030 36

Julio-César García and Rosa-Helena Bustos
The Genetic Diagnosis of Neurodegenerative Diseases and Therapeutic Perspectives
Reprinted from: *Brain Sci.* **2018**, *8*, 222, doi:10.3390/brainsci8120222 51

Edward Botsford, Jayan George and Ellen E. Buckley
Parkinson's Disease and Metal Storage Disorders: A Systematic Review
Reprinted from: *Brain Sci.* **2018**, *8*, 194, doi:10.3390/brainsci8110194 69

About the Special Issue Editor

Alisdair McNeill, Dr, received his MBChB (Hons) from Edinburgh University in 2004, and obtained his MRCP (UK) in 2007. He undertook Medical SHO training in Newcastle-upon-Tyne and Edinburgh, Clinical Genetics SpR training in the West Midlands, and an MRC Clinical Research Training Fellowship at UCL. His research interests are focused on the genetic causes of neurological disorders in both children and adults. McNeill is identifying new ways of phenotyping patients in order to improve diagnosis and disease monitoring, for example, through using patient-wearable movement sensors (collaboration with INSIGNEO) in adults with neurological disorders and 3-dimensional facial image analysis (collaboration with Prof Peter Hammond, Oxford) in children with chromosome microdeletions. He is also interested in studying variants of uncertain significance as identified in clinical genetics testing, and resolving their pathogenicity through clinical phenotyping and in vitro studies.

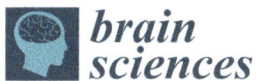

Editorial

Editorial for *Brain Sciences* Special Issue: "Diagnosis of Neurogenetic Disorders: Contribution of Next-Generation Sequencing and Deep Phenotyping"

Alisdair McNeill

Department of Neuroscience, University of Sheffield, 385a Glossop Road, Sheffield S10 2HQ, UK; a.mcneill@sheffield.ac.uk

Received: 11 March 2019; Accepted: 19 March 2019; Published: 26 March 2019

In this Special Issue we bring together papers demonstrating the need for both detailed genomic and phenotypic studies to aid our scientific and clinical understanding of neurogenetic disorders. Genomic techniques such as genome and exome sequencing are vital tools for diagnosing rare neurogenetic disorders and identifying novel causal genes [1,2]. In this Special Issue, Gardner and colleagues [3] utilise genomic techniques to identify a series of individuals with brain malformations due to the recurrent *TUBA1A p.Arg2His* variant. This paper also describes the detailed phenotyping required to aid in the interpretation of novel genomic variants. Variants in *GBA1*, the gene causing Gaucher Disease (GD), are associated with an increased risk of Parkinson's Disease (PD) [4,5]. Gatto and colleagues review this important area and describe how simple clinical observations helped begin the identification of this important risk factor for PD [6]. Genomic techniques are crucial for the diagnosis of neurogenetic disorders [7]. Garcia and Bustos [8] review the impact of such techniques for both the diagnosis of neurogenetic diseases and increasing our scientific understanding of these disorders. It is only through the co-development of both novel genomic and phenotypic assessments that we will be able to fully understand the pathogenesis of neurogenetic disorders and identify novel treatments.

Conflicts of Interest: The author declares no conflict of interest.

References

1. Hempel, A.; Pagnamenta, A.T.; Blyth, M.; Mansour, S.; McConnell, V.; Kou, I.; Ikegawa, S.; Tsurusaki, Y.; Matsumoto, N.; Lo-Castro, A.; et al. Deletions and de novo mutations of SOX11 are associated with a neurodevelopmental disorder with features of Coffin-Siris syndrome. *J. Med. Genet.* **2016**, *53*, 152–162. [CrossRef] [PubMed]
2. Blanchet, P.; Bebin, M.; Bruet, S.; Cooper, G.M.; Thompson, M.L.; Duban-Bedu, B.; Gerard, B.; Piton, A.; Suckno, S.; Deshpande, C.; et al. MYT1L mutations cause intellectual disability and variable obesity by dysregulating gene expression and development of the neuroendocrine hypothalamus. *Plos Genet.* **2017**, *13*, e1006957. [CrossRef] [PubMed]
3. Gardner, J.F.; Cushion, T.D.; Niotakis, G.; Olson, H.E.; Grant, P.E.; Scott, R.H.; Stoodley, N.; Cohen, J.S.; Naidu, S.; Attie-Bitach, T.; Bonnières, M.; Boutaud, L.; Encha-Razavi, F.; Palmer-Smith, S.M.; Mugalaasi, H.; Mullins, J.G.L.; Pilz, D.T.; Fry, A.E. Clinical and Functional Characterization of the Recurrent TUBA1A p.(Arg2His) Mutation. *Brain Sci.* **2018**, *8*, 145. [CrossRef] [PubMed]
4. McNeill, A.; Duran, R.; Proukakis, C.; Bras, J.; Hughes, D.; Mehta, A.; Hardy, J.; Wood, N.W.; Wood, A.H.V. Hyposmia and cognitive impairment in Gaucher disease patients and carriers. *Mov. Disord.* **2012**, *27*, 526–532. [CrossRef] [PubMed]
5. McNeill, A.; Duran, R.; Hughes, D.A.; Mehta, A.; Schapira, A.H. A clinical and family history study of Parkinson's disease in heterozygous glucocerebrosidase mutation carriers. *J. Neurol. Neurosurg. Psych.* **2012**, *83*, 853–854. [CrossRef] [PubMed]

6. Gatto, E.M.; Da Prat, G.; Etcheverry, J.L.; Drelichman, G.; Cesarini, M. Parkinsonisms and Glucocerebrosidase Deficiency: A Comprehensive Review for Molecular and Cellular Mechanism of Glucocerebrosidase Deficiency. *Brain Sci.* **2019**, *9*, 30. [CrossRef] [PubMed]
7. Majewski, J.; Schwartzentruber, J.; Lalonde, E.; Montpetit, A.; Jabado, N. What can exome sequencing do for you? *J. Med. Genet.* **2011**, *48*, 580–589. [CrossRef] [PubMed]
8. García, J.-C.; Bustos, R.-H. The Genetic Diagnosis of Neurodegenerative Diseases and Therapeutic Perspectives. *Brain Sci.* **2018**, *8*, 222. [CrossRef] [PubMed]

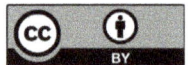

© 2019 by the author. Licensee MDPI, Basel, Switzerland. This article is an open access article distributed under the terms and conditions of the Creative Commons Attribution (CC BY) license (http://creativecommons.org/licenses/by/4.0/).

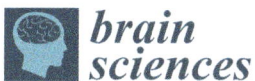 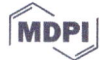

Article

Clinical and Functional Characterization of the Recurrent TUBA1A p.(Arg2His) Mutation

Jennifer F. Gardner [1,†], Thomas D. Cushion [2,†], Georgios Niotakis [3], Heather E. Olson [4], P. Ellen Grant [5], Richard H. Scott [6], Neil Stoodley [7], Julie S. Cohen [8], Sakkubai Naidu [8,9,10], Tania Attie-Bitach [11,12], Maryse Bonnières [11], Lucile Boutaud [11,12], Férechté Encha-Razavi [11], Sheila M. Palmer-Smith [1], Hood Mugalaasi [1], Jonathan G. L. Mullins [13], Daniela T. Pilz [2,14] and Andrew E. Fry [1,2,*]

1. Institute of Medical Genetics, University Hospital of Wales, Cardiff CF14 4XW, UK; jennifer.gardner@wales.nhs.uk (J.F.G.); sheila.palmer-smith@wales.nhs.uk (S.M.P.-S.); hood.mugalaasi@wales.nhs.uk (H.M.)
2. Division of Cancer and Genetics, School of Medicine, Cardiff University, Cardiff CF14 4XN, UK; cushiont@cardiff.ac.uk (T.D.C.); pilzdt@cardiff.ac.uk (D.T.P.)
3. Paediatrics Department, Venizelion Hospital, Knossos Ave, P.O. Box 44, Heraklion, 714 09 Crete, Greece; niotakisg@yahoo.gr
4. Epilepsy Genetics Program, Department of Neurology, Division of Epilepsy and Clinical Neurophysiology, Boston Children's Hospital, Boston, MA 02115, USA; heather.olson@childrens.harvard.edu
5. Fetal-Neonatal Neuroimaging and Developmental Science Center, Boston Children's Hospital, Harvard Medical School, Boston, MA 02115, USA; ellen.grant@childrens.harvard.edu
6. Clinical Genetics Unit, Great Ormond Street Hospital for Children NHS Trust, Great Ormond Street, London WC1N 3JH, UK; richard.scott@genomicsengland.co.uk
7. Department of Neuroradiology, North Bristol NHS Trust, Frenchay Hospital, Bristol BS16 1LE, UK; neilstoodley@doctors.org.uk
8. Division of Neurogenetics, Hugo W. Moser Research Institute, Kennedy Krieger Institute, Baltimore, MD 21205, USA; cohenju@kennedykrieger.org (J.S.C.); naidu@kennedykrieger.org (S.N.)
9. Department of Neurology, The Johns Hopkins Hospital, Baltimore, Maryland, MD 21287, USA
10. Department of Pediatrics, The Johns Hopkins Hospital, Baltimore, Maryland, MD 21287, USA
11. Unité d'Embryofœtopathologie, Service d'Histologie Embryologie Cytogénétique, Hôpital Necker-Enfants Malades, Assistance Publique Hôpitaux de Paris (APHP), 75004 Paris, France; tania.attie@inserm.fr (T.A.-B.); maryse.bonniere-darcy@aphp.fr (M.B.); lucile.boutaud@gmail.com (L.B.); ferechte.razavi@aphp.fr (F.E.-R.)
12. Institut Imagine, INSERM U1163, Université Paris Descartes, Sorbonne Paris Cite, 75006 Paris, France
13. Institute of Life Science, Swansea University Medical School, Swansea SA2 8PP, UK; j.g.l.mullins@swansea.ac.uk
14. Department of Clinical Genetics, West of Scotland Regional Genetics Service, Queen Elizabeth University Hospital, Glasgow G51 4TF, UK
* Correspondence: fryae@cardiff.ac.uk; Tel.: +44-292-074-3151
† These authors contributed equally to this work.

Received: 30 May 2018; Accepted: 17 July 2018; Published: 7 August 2018

Abstract: The *TUBA1A* gene encodes tubulin alpha-1A, a protein that is highly expressed in the fetal brain. Alpha- and beta-tubulin subunits form dimers, which then co-assemble into microtubule polymers: dynamic, scaffold-like structures that perform key functions during neurogenesis, neuronal migration, and cortical organisation. Mutations in *TUBA1A* have been reported to cause a range of brain malformations. We describe four unrelated patients with the same de novo missense mutation in *TUBA1A*, c.5G>A, p.(Arg2His), as found by next generation sequencing. Detailed comparison revealed similar brain phenotypes with mild variability. Shared features included developmental delay, microcephaly, hypoplasia of the cerebellar vermis, dysplasia or thinning of the corpus callosum, small pons, and dysmorphic basal ganglia. Two of the patients had bilateral perisylvian polymicrogyria. We examined the effects of the p.(Arg2His) mutation by computer-based protein structure modelling and heterologous expression in HEK-293 cells.

The results suggest the mutation subtly impairs microtubule function, potentially by affecting inter-dimer interaction. Based on its sequence context, c.5G>A is likely to be a common recurrent mutation. We propose that the subtle functional effects of p.(Arg2His) may allow for other factors (such as genetic background or environmental conditions) to influence phenotypic outcome, thus explaining the mild variability in clinical manifestations.

Keywords: *TUBA1A*; tubulin; p.(Arg2His), R2H; tubulinopathy; polymicrogyria; cerebellar hypoplasia

1. Introduction

TUBA1A is a highly-conserved gene with few changes among eukaryotes and few polymorphic variants in human populations. *TUBA1A* encodes the tubulin alpha-1A chain, a protein that is highly-expressed in the cerebral cortex, hippocampus, cerebellum, and brainstem of the developing fetal brain, with a decrease in postnatal and adult stages [1,2]. Alpha- and beta-tubulin subunits form dimers that coassemble into microtubules. Microtubules are dynamic polymers that perform a range of mechanical tasks within the cell. As major components of the mitotic spindle, microtubules control division of neuronal progenitors to produce neurons. In turn, they generate the push-and-pull forces that are required for the migration of primitive neurons, from deep proliferative areas to the cortical plate. Subsequently, bundles of stable and polarised microtubule polymers generate long axons facilitating cortical organisation and synaptic connectivity.

TUBA1A was the first tubulin gene to be associated with human brain malformations [3]. Mutations in *TUBA1A* have been reported in patients with a range of brain malformations, including lissencephaly, microlissencephaly, polymicrogyria, and simplified gyri [4–6]. They have also been reported in patients with hydranencephaly-like dysplasias, cerebral palsy, and autistic spectrum disorders [7–9]. *TUBA1A* mutations (as with other tubulinopathies) are often associated with hypoplasia/agenesis of the corpus callosum, hypoplasia/dysplasia of the cerebellum, and dysmorphic basal ganglia [5,6]. Common clinical features in *TUBA1A* patients include microcephaly, intellectual disability, motor impairment, and epilepsy. Mutations in several other tubulin genes have been reported in patients with brain malformations including TUBB2B [10], TUBB3 [11,12], TUBB [13], TUBB2A [14], and *TUBG1* [15]. However, *TUBA1A* mutations remain the most common cause of tubulin-related brain malformations, with over 60 mutations being described to date [6]. Most disease-causing *TUBA1A* mutations are de novo, although familial recurrence due to parental somatic mosaicism has been reported [4,16].

Pathogenic *TUBA1A* mutations have been found distributed throughout the gene. A handful of recurrent *TUBA1A* mutations have been reported. These include the p.(Arg402His) mutation, which has been reported in at least five patients and is associated with classic lissencephaly [3,17]. Similarly, the recurrent p.(Arg264Cys) mutation has been found in several patients and is typically associated with central pachygyria [3,18,19]. Few genotype-phenotype correlations have been reported for *TUBA1A*. However, the phenotypic effects of a specific recurrent mutation are generally consistent. Alpha-tubulin must fold in a precise way and present specific shapes and charges on its surface to interact with other proteins (e.g., beta-tubulin subunits, microtubule binding proteins) and to correctly handle and hydrolyse guanosine-5'-triphosphate (GTP). Many *TUBA1A* mutations have been shown to disrupt protein folding and/or heterodimer formation, resulting in either a reduced yield or reduced stability [20].

During the clinical diagnostic work-up of two unrelated patients with developmental delay and brain abnormalities, we identified the same mutation, c.5G>A, p.(Arg2His), in *TUBA1A*. To define the clinical consequences of this mutation, we collected detailed phenotype information from both patients and two additional patients that were previously reported in the literature [21–23]. We examined the functional impact of the mutation by in vitro microtubule studies and computer-based protein structure modeling.

2. Materials and Methods

2.1. Patients

Patients 1 and 2 were diagnosed during routine clinical diagnostic work-ups. Patient 1 underwent testing with a 12-gene polymicrogyria sequencing panel (targets enriched by Agilent SureSelect system, followed by Illumina sequencing) in the United States. Patient 2 had testing with a 40 gene cortical malformation gene panel (HaploPlex target enrichment system followed by Illumina sequencing) in the United Kingdom. The mutations in Patients 1 and 2 were confirmed and shown to be de novo by Sanger sequencing in the patient and both parents. Patient 3 underwent trio-based whole exome sequencing (WES) as a part of their routine clinical diagnostic work-up in the United States [21,23]. The approach to analysis and filtering of the WES data has previously been described [21]. No other candidate variants were identified in the patient. Patient 4 underwent targeted sequencing of a panel of 423 genes that are associated with corpus callosum anomalies in France [22]. The approach to analysis and filtering of this panel has previously been described [24,25]. No other candidate variants were identified in the patient. Consent was obtained from the parents of all the participants for publication. The genomic location of the mutation is chr12:g.49580615C>T (GRCh37/hg19), rs587784491. Coding and protein positions of *TUBA1A* mutations are based on GenBank accession codes NM_006009.3 (ENST00000301071.7) and NP_006000.2, respectively.

2.2. Homology Modelling

Structural predictions of wild-type and mutant TUBA1A protein subunits were generated while using a previously-described homology modeling pipeline [26]. This approach uses the solved structure of a homologous template to predict the folding of a target sequence. The target sequence was wild-type TUBA1A (NP_006000.2). The template used was the crystal structure of Tubulin alpha-1B from *Bos taurus* (Protein Data Bank (PDB): 4I4T) [27], which shares 99% sequencing identity with human TUBA1A. Microtubule architecture was based on a previously published template (PDB: 2XRP) [28]. Homology modelling was performed by MODELLER (version 9.17) [29]. Structural models were viewed and analysed while using the UCSF Chimera software (version 1.12) [30,31].

2.3. Expression Construct Mutagenesis and Cell Culture

A C-terminally FLAG-tagged wild-type TUBA1A expression construct (pRK5-TUBA1A-C-FLAG) was modified to generate TUBA1A-R2H by site-directed mutagenesis using the QuikChange mutagenesis kit (Stratagene, La Jolla, CA, USA). HEK-293 cells were cultured in Dulbecco's modified Eagle's media (ThermoFisher, Waltham, MA, USA, catalogue number 41966029), supplemented with 10% fetal calf serum (ThermoFisher, 10500056) and 1% penicillin/streptomycin (ThermoFisher, 15070063), as previously described [14].

2.4. Immunocytochemistry

HEK-293 cells were cultured in Dulbecco's modified Eagle's media (ThermoFisher, 41966029). supplemented with 10% fetal calf serum (ThermoFisher, 10500056) and 1% penicillin/streptomycin (ThermoFisher, 15070063) and incubated at 37 °C 5% CO_2. Cells were seeded onto poly-D-Lysine (Sigma-Aldrich, St. Louis, MO, USA, P6407) pre-coated 13 mm glass coverslips. After 24 h, the cells were transfected with either wild-type or mutant expression constructs using Lipofectamine 2000 (ThermoFisher, 11668030). Twenty-four hours post-transfection, the cells were fixed with methanol at −20 °C for five minutes. Fixed cells were blocked with blocking buffer (phosphate-buffered saline (PBS) with 2% Bovine Serum Albumin (BSA; Sigma-Aldrich, B4287) and 0.5% Triton (Sigma-Aldrich, T8787)) for 30 min at room temperature (23 °C). Cells were immunostained with rabbit anti-FLAG

(Sigma-Aldrich, F7425; 1:500) and mouse anti-alpha-tubulin (Sigma-Aldrich, T6199; 1:750) diluted in PBS with 2% BSA and 0.1% Triton for one hour at room temperature. Primary antibodies were aspirated, cells washed three times with PBS, and incubated with AlexaFluor[568]-conjugated goat anti-rabbit (ThermoFisher, A11011) and AlexaFluor[488]-conjugated goat anti-mouse (ThermoFisher, A11011) secondary antibodies for 30 minutes at room temperature, and protected from light from this point onwards. Cells were rinsed with PBS, mounted onto glass slides with ProLong Gold mounting medium (ThermoFisher, P10144) and stored at 4 °C until examined by confocal microscopy (Zeiss Axioscope).

2.5. Predicting the Probability of TUBA1A Substitutions

The genomic DNA sequence of the *TUBA1A* gene (based on transcript ENST00000301071.7) was obtained from the Ensembl Genome Browser [32]. A sliding window was implemented using a Perl script. For each 7-nucleotide window the script recorded the position and base of the central nucleotide. The heptanucleotide sequence was then looked up in the data from [33] (Supplementary Table 7 from that paper). The substitution probabilities for changing the central nucleotide to each of the three alternative bases were taken (averaging African, Asian, and European values). The cDNA and protein consequences of each substitution were derived using Mutalyzer [34,35]. Predicted substitution probabilities were obtained for all coding positions, introns (±20 base pairs flanking exons), and 5' and 3' untranslated regions (±20 base pairs).

3. Results

3.1. Clinical Features of Patients with the p.(Arg2His) Mutation

We identified two unrelated patients (Patients 1 and 2) with the same *TUBA1A* missense mutation, c.5G>A, p.(Arg2His). A search of the literature found reports of two additional patients with the p.(Arg2His) mutation (Patients 3 and 4) [21–23]. Only brief descriptions of the two published subjects were previously available. We obtained detailed clinical information from the four individuals (Table 1, detailed case reports are provided in the Supplementary Material). All four mutations were de novo. Consistent features in the living patients were developmental delay and microcephaly. MRI brain images from Patients 1–3 were available for review (Figure 1). The images demonstrated the hypoplasia and dysplasia of the cerebellar vermis (3/3), hypoplasia or dysgenesis of the corpus callosum (3/3), and dysmorphic basal ganglia (3/3). Patient 1 had bilateral perisylvian polymicrogyria. The pons of all three patients was small, particularly affecting the belly of the pons.

Patient 4 was a fetus terminated at 36 weeks gestation. Post-mortem examination of Patient 4 found a small brain (weight on 5th centile) with shortening of the corpus callosum and cerebellar hypoplasia (Figure 2A,B). Neuropathology examination found bilateral perisylvian polymicrogyria (Figure 2C–E). At the supratentorial level, callosal fibers and corticospinal tracts (CST) were hypoplastic. The brainstem was shortened and dysmorphic, displaying a Z-shaped kink. At the level of the cerebral peduncles, the CST were present but reduced in size. The pons was reduced in size in its basilar part. In the pons the CST were present at the junction with the peduncles but showed a chaotic pattern in between the pontine nuclei. The transverse pontine fibers were also reduced, and associated with cerebellar heterotopias and hypoplastic deep nuclei. At the level of the medulla, the pyramids were present but hypoplastic. The inferior olivary nuclei were also reduced in size. Neuronal heterotopia of the olivary nuclei was noted. At the cervical spinal cord level, crossing CST were absent. Cerebellar foliation was normal, but lamination was impaired with rare and misaligned Purkinje cells.

Table 1. Clinical features of patients with the recurrent p.(Arg2His) TUBA1A mutation.

Patient	1	2	3	4 (fetus)
Sex	Male	Male	Male	Male
OFC at Birth	30 cm (−3.6 SD)	34 cm (−0.9 SD)	33 cm (−1.7 SD)	n/a
Age at last review	4 years	32 months	37 months	TOP at 36 weeks gestation
Last OFC	45 cm (−4.9 SD)	43 cm (−5.9 SD)	45 cm (−4.6 SD)	n/a
Developmental delay	Moderate	Severe	Moderate	n/a
Seizures	Yes (onset at 3 years)	Yes (onset at 12 months)	No	n/a
Cerebral cortex	Bilateral perisylvian polymicrogyria	Normal	Normal	Bilateral perisylvian polymicrogyria
White matter	Reduced	Reduced	Reduced	n/k
Corpus callosum	Partial agenesis	Thin	Thin	Short, no rostrum
Basal ganglia	Dysmorphic, prominent	Dysmorphic, prominent	Dysmorphic, prominent	n/k
Cerebellum	Hypoplasia and dysplasia of vermis	Hypoplasia and dysplasia of vermis	Hypoplasia and dysplasia of vermis	Hypoplasia, Impaired lamination, rare and misaligned Purkinje
Brainstem	Small pons	Small pons	Small pons	Neuronal heterotopia of olivary nuclei and hypoplastic pyramids

Key: n/a/k = not applicable/known; OFC = occipital frontal circumference; PMG = polymicrogyria; SD = standard deviations; TOP = termination of pregnancy.

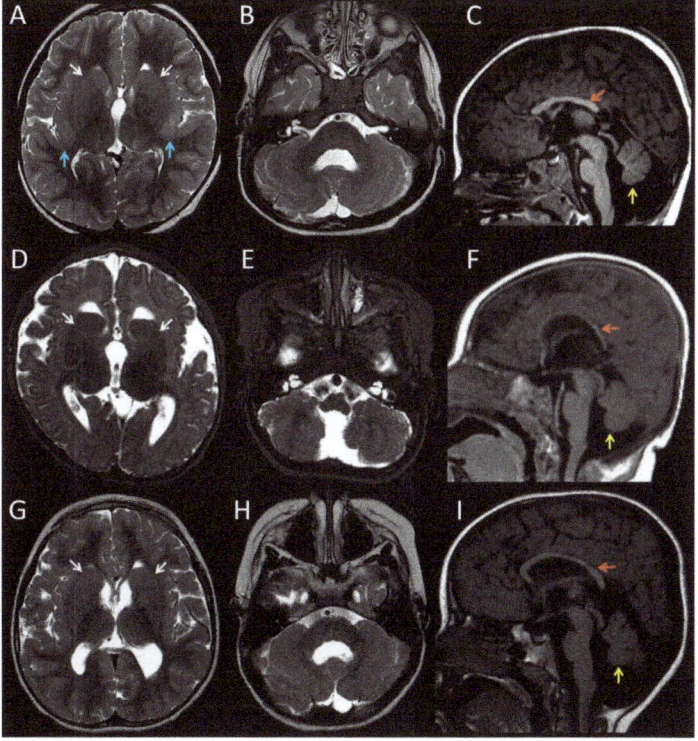

Figure 1. Magnetic resonance images from patients with the recurrent p.(Arg2His) TUBA1A mutation. T2-weighted axial and T1-weighted midline sagittal brain images for Patient 1 at age three years (**A–C**), Patient 2 at age six months (**D–F**), and Patient 3 at age 19 months (**G–I**). The images demonstrate hypoplasia and dysplasia of the cerebellar vermis (yellow arrows), thinning or partial agenesis of the corpus callosum (red arrows), globular basal ganglia with incomplete formation of the anterior limb internal capsule (white arrows), and bilateral perisylvian polymicrogyria (blue arrows). The pons is similar in size to the midbrain which suggests the pons is relatively small (**C,F,I**).

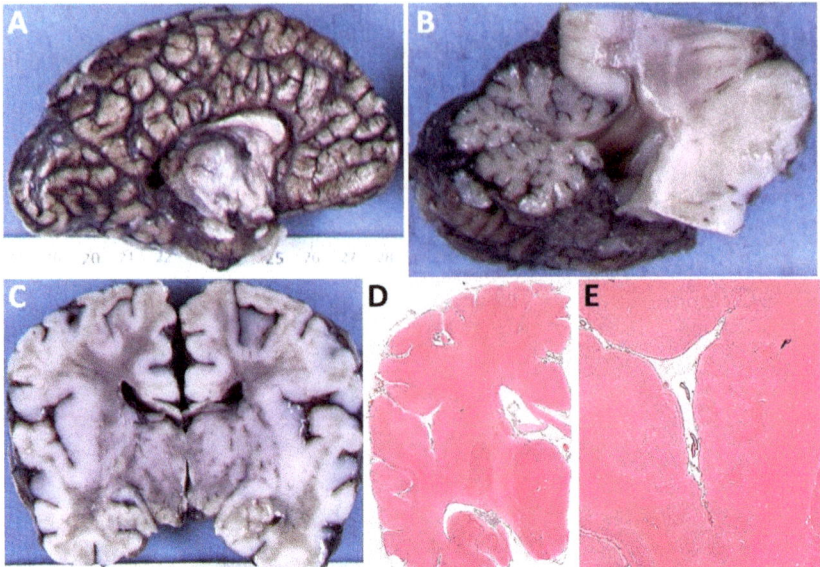

Figure 2. Neuropathology from Patient 4. (**A**) The medial aspect of right cerebral hemisphere showing a thin corpus callosom with absent rostrum. (**B**) Midline sagittal section of brain stem and cerebellum showing mild hypoplasia of the cerebellar vermis. (**C**) Coronal section of the cerebral hemispheres. The corpus callosum is thinned and there is thickening of the cortex around the sylvian fissures. (**D**) Stained section of the right cerebral hemisphere revealing abnormal folding of the cortical ribbon around the sylvian fissure. (**E**) A magnified view of (**D**) demonstrating polymicrogyria around the sylvian fissure.

3.2. Modelling the Structural Effects of p.Arg2His

The Arg2 residue of TUBA1A is highly conserved across species and tubulin isoforms (Figure S1). The p.(Arg2His) variant is not present in gnomAD and multiple in silico prediction tools suggest it is deleterious (Table S1). However, the physicochemical difference between arginine and histidine is relatively small (Grantham difference 29) with both of the residues having positively-charged side chains. The c.5G>A change is predicted to have minimal effects on the splicing at the adjacent splice acceptor site (Figure S2). When incorporated into polymerised microtubule, the N-terminus of alpha-tubulin is positioned near the inter-dimer interface, between the alpha-tubulin subunit of one heterodimer and the beta subunit of the next heterodimer. To study the effects of p.Arg2His on the three-dimensional structure of the protein, we compared wild-type and mutant TUBA1A by modelling the alpha/beta-tubulin heterodimer (Figure 3A,B) (the protein variant is given here without brackets as we know the amino acid sequence in a simulation). The effects of the mutation were mild. No predicted hydrogen bonding was lost or gained between the alpha- and beta-tubulin subunits as a result of p.Arg2His. A hydrogen bond between Arg2 and the highly-conserved Cys4 residue within TUBA1A was lost. In addition, new bonds between Glu3, and both Asn50 and Thr130 were predicted to form as a result of the substitution. Additional conformational changes were predicted to occur in a loop region (Asp38 to Asn51, Figure 3B), which may affect interactions between heterodimers.

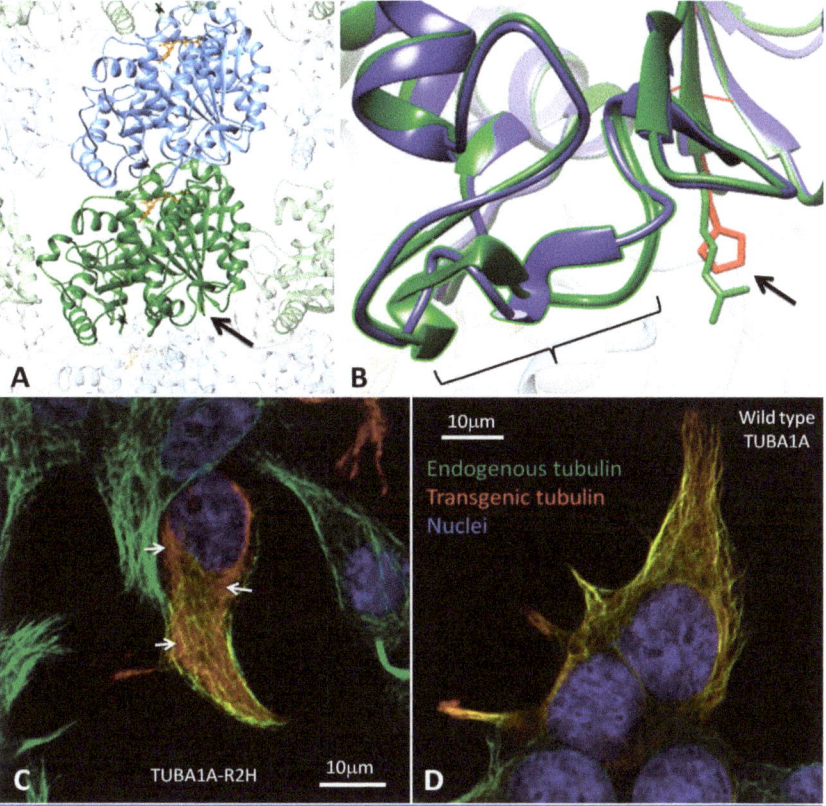

Figure 3. In silico modelling and in vitro functional analysis of the p.(Arg2His) mutation. (**A**) Ribbon models of alpha-tubulin (green) and beta-tubulin (blue) subunits aligned in a microtubule polymer. The position of Arg2 is shown (arrow) close to the inter-dimer interface (between alpha-tubulin and the beta-tubulin of an adjacent heterodimer). The mutation is on the opposite side of TUBA1A from the binding site of guanosine-5′-triphosphate (GTP, orange). (**B**) A close-up view of the Arg2 residue (arrow) with the mutant (purple ribbon, red side chain) and wild type (green ribbon and side chain) proteins superimposed. Only mild confirmation changes are predicted around the Arg2 residue. However, additional conformational changes are predicted between residues 38 and 51 (bracket). These may affect the interaction between heterodimers. (**C**) HEK-293 cells expressing FLAG-tagged TUBA1A-R2H. The cells are stained with DAPI (4′,6-diamidino-2-phenylindole, blue), anti-FLAG- (red), and anti-alpha-tubulin (green) antibodies. The microtubules appear yellow due to the colocalisation of endogenous (green) and FLAG-tagged transgenic (red) tubulin. The arrows indicate diffuse patches of transgenic mutant tubulin (red) in the cytoplasm between the microtubules. (**D**) Control cells expressing FLAG-tagged wild-type TUBA1A have less staining for the transgenic tubulin in the cytoplasm between the microtubules.

3.3. Heterologous Expression of TUBA1A-R2H in HEK-293 cells

TUBA1A containing the p.(Arg2His) mutation (TUBA1A-R2H) was expressed in cultured HEK-293 cells. TUBA1A-R2H incorporated into the microtubule polymer network (Figure 3C), suggesting that it successfully folds and dimerises with endogenous beta-tubulin. However, in comparison to wild-type TUBA1A (Figure 3D), there was a slight increase in the proportion of the mutant FLAG-tagged protein seen unpolymerised within the cytosol. This suggests the mutation subtly alters the function (folding, dimerisation, or coassembly) of the subunit, but that once incorporated the dynamics of the mutant subunit are similar to wild type.

3.4. Substitution Probability of Recurrent TUBA1A Mutations

The observation of p.(Arg2His) on four separate occasions suggested that it was a common recurrent *TUBA1A* mutation. However, we noted that p.(Arg2His) had not been reported in previous large tubulinopathy cohorts [6]. In contrast, several *TUBA1A* mutations have been found recurrently in tubulinopathy patients. Examples include p.(Arg214His) [6,36], p.(Arg264Cys) [3,18,19], p.(Arg390Cys) [17,37], p.(Arg402His) [3,17,38,39], p.(Arg402Cys) [17,19], and p.(Arg422His) [17,18,40]. This made us wonder whether p.(Arg2His) had a lower mutation rate than the other recurrent *TUBA1A* mutations or whether it was just ascertained less frequently. We observed that the recurrent mutations all occurred at CpG sites, which are prone to spontaneous deamination (CGx is the codon for arginine). This highlighted that sequence context was likely to be an important factor. To predict the substitution rates at these sites and to compare them with the rest of *TUBA1A*, we estimated the probability of all possible single-base substitutions in *TUBA1A* based on heptanucleotide context (target position and three flanking nucleotides either side). Heptanucleotide context has been shown to explain >81% of variability in substitution probabilities [33]. We found the seven recurrent *TUBA1A* mutations all ranked in the top 1% for substitution probability. The p.(Arg2His) mutation was the second highest in the group (ranking 7th out of 4548 possible substitutions) (Table S2). These results suggest p.(Arg2His) has a mutation rate that is similar to other recurrent *TUBA1A* mutations. The lack of observations in previous tubulinopathy cohorts may therefore reflect differences in ascertainment.

4. Discussion

In this report, we describe four patients with the TUBA1A p.(Arg2His) mutation. The patients had similar phenotypes with mild variability. Shared features included developmental delay, microcephaly, hypoplasia, and dysplasia of the cerebellar vermis, dysplasia or thinning of the corpus callosum, and dysmorphic basal ganglia. The pons tended to be small, disproportionally affecting the belly of the pons. We suspect the pons is dyspastic (i.e., abnormally developed) as well as small. Histopathological abnormalities of the pons were noted in patient 4. Two of the patients had bilateral perisylvian polymicrogyria. These features are typical of a tubulinopathy spectrum disorder [6]. Our findings suggest that p.(Arg2His) is a common recurrent *TUBA1A* mutation. Tubulinopathy patients are often ascertained due to cortical malformations (e.g., the classical lissencephaly associated with the recurrent p.(Arg402His) mutation)). In contrast, p.(Arg2His) does not cause an extensive cortical malformation. This may explain why p.(Arg2His) has not been observed in previous tubulinopathy cohorts [6].

Phenotypic variability that is associated with recurrent *TUBA1A* mutations has previously been noted. For example, the p.(Arg390Cys) mutation was first reported in a patient with mild gyral simplification, complete agenesis of the corpus callosum, and cerebellar hypoplasia [17]. It was subsequently reported in a patient with asymmetrical perisylvian polymicrogyria, hypoplasia of the corpus callosum, dysplastic cerebellar vermis, dysmorphic basal ganglia, and severe hypoplasia of brainstem [37]. Similarly, p.(Arg214His) was initially reported in a fetus with central polymicrogyria-like cortical dysplasia, complete agenesis of the corpus callosum, and normal cerebellum [6]. It was then reported in a patient with diffuse irregular gyration and sulcation of the cortex, partial agenesis of the corpus callosum, hypoplasia of the cerebellar vermis, and globular thalami [36]. As with p.(Arg2His), these descriptions suggest variability, but with overlap in key elements of the phenotype (abnormalities of the cortex, corpus callosum, cerebellum, and basal ganglia). Some of the variability may be due to differences in the interpretation of the brain imaging. However, differences in genetic background, environmental factors, or random chance may also contribute. Oegema et al. [36] found that p.(Arg214His) caused only a mild functional deficit (incorporating into microtubule polymers at comparable levels to wild type but at a reduced rate) and subtle predicted structural effects. Mutations with relatively mild functional effects (such as p.(Arg214His) or p.(Arg2His)) may allow for other factors to influence phenotype outcome.

Mutations of the homologous Arg2 residue in other tubulin isoforms have been linked to human disease phenotypes. TUBB8 is the main beta-tubulin of oocytes. The p.(Arg2Lys) mutation in TUBB8 has been found to cause arrest of oocyte meosis [41]. The mutation is thought to affect folding of the protein as well as the assembly and stability of heterodimers. The p.(Arg2Met) mutation in TUBB8 has also been shown to cause arrest of oocyte maturation [42,43]. TUBB4A is a brain-expressed beta-tubulin isoform. A p.(Arg2Gly) mutation in TUBB4A has been identified in a family with dystonia type 4 ('Whispering dysphonia') [44,45]. TUBB4A p.(Arg2Trp) and p.(Arg2Gln) have been reported to cause hypomyelination with atrophy of the basal ganglia and cerebellum [46,47]. The Arg2 of TUBB4A is part of the MREI (Met-Arg-Glu-Ile) 'auto-regulatory' domain, which is involved in controlling the amount of the beta-tubulin produced by the cell. In addition, these mutations disrupt a salt bridge Arg2 forms with Asp249 in TUBB4A [48]. This salt bridge is not predicted to occur in TUBA1A as the homologous residues are further apart.

5. Conclusions

We have shown that the *TUBA1A* c.5G>A, p.(Arg2His) mutation causes cortical, callosal, and cerebellar abnormalities that are typical of tubulinopathy-associated brain malformations. Based on its sequence context (and observation in four unrelated patients), c.5G>A is likely to be a common recurrent mutation in *TUBA1A*. Our functional and computer modelling results suggest that p.(Arg2His) has subtle effects on microtubule function, possibly acting at the inter-dimer interface. We propose that the subtle functional effects of the mutation may allow for other factors (e.g., genetic background, environmental conditions, or random chance) to modulate outcome, explaining the mild phenotypic variability observed.

Supplementary Materials: The following are available online at http://www.mdpi.com/2076-3425/8/8/145/s1, Supplementary File 1 containing Figure S1: Sequences from orthologs and paralogs of TUBA1A demonstrating conservation of the Arg2 residue, Figure S2: In silico RNA splicing prediction reports, Table S1: In silico predictions and population data, and the detailed clinical descriptions of the four patients with the TUBA1A p.(Arg2His) mutation; Supplementary File 2 containing Table S2: The substitution probabilities for 4548 possible substitutions in the *TUBA1A* gene based on heptanucleotide sequence context.

Author Contributions: Conceptualization, T.D.C. and A.E.F.; Formal analysis, T.D.C. and A.E.F.; Investigation, J.F.G., T.D.C., G.N., H.E.O., P.E.G., R.H.S., N.S., J.S.C., S.N., T.A.-B., M.B., L.B., F.E.-R., S.M.P.-S., H.M., D.T.P. and A.E.F.; Software, T.D.C., J.G.L.M. and A.E.F.; Writing-original draft, J.F.G., T.D.C. and A.E.F.; Writing-review & editing, G.N., H.E.O., P.E.G., R.H.S., N.S., J.S.C., S.N., T.A.-B., M.B., L.B., F.E.-R., S.M.P.-S., H.M., J.G.L.M. and D.T.P.

Funding: The project was supported by the Wales Gene Park and the Wales Epilepsy Research Network.

Acknowledgments: The authors would like to thank the patients, families, clinicians and scientists who contributed to this work. We would like to thank Mark I. Rees (College of Medicine, Swansea University) for donating the wild-type pRK5-TUBA1A-C-FLAG construct.

Conflicts of Interest: The authors declare no conflict of interest.

References

1. Gloster, A.; Wu, W.; Speelman, A.; Weiss, S.; Causing, C.; Pozniak, C.; Reynolds, B.; Chang, E.; Toma, J.G.; Miller, F.D. The T alpha 1 alpha-tubulin promoter specifies gene expression as a function of neuronal growth and regeneration in transgenic mice. *J. Neurosci.* **1994**, *14*, 7319–7330. [CrossRef] [PubMed]
2. Bamji, S.X.; Miller, F.D. Comparison of the expression of a T alpha 1:nlacZ transgene and T alpha 1 alpha-tubulin mRNA in the mature central nervous system. *J. Comp. Neurol.* **1996**, *374*, 52–69. [CrossRef]
3. Keays, D.A.; Tian, G.; Poirier, K.; Huang, G.-J.; Siebold, C.; Cleak, J.; Oliver, P.L.; Fray, M.; Harvey, R.J.; Molnár, Z.; et al. Mutations in alpha-tubulin cause abnormal neuronal migration in mice and lissencephaly in humans. *Cell* **2007**, *128*, 45–57. [CrossRef] [PubMed]

4. Jansen, A.C.; Oostra, A.; Desprechins, B.; De Vlaeminck, Y.; Verhelst, H.; Régal, L.; Verloo, P.; Bockaert, N.; Keymolen, K.; Seneca, S.; et al. TUBA1A mutations: from isolated lissencephaly to familial polymicrogyria. *Neurology* **2011**, *76*, 988–992. [CrossRef] [PubMed]
5. Cushion, T.D.; Dobyns, W.B.; Mullins, J.G.L.; Stoodley, N.; Chung, S.-K.; Fry, A.E.; Hehr, U.; Gunny, R.; Aylsworth, A.S.; Prabhakar, P.; et al. Overlapping cortical malformations and mutations in TUBB2B and TUBA1A. *Brain* **2013**, *136*, 536–548. [CrossRef] [PubMed]
6. Bahi-Buisson, N.; Poirier, K.; Fourniol, F.; Saillour, Y.; Valence, S.; Lebrun, N.; Hully, M.; Bianco, C.F.; Boddaert, N.; Elie, C.; et al. The wide spectrum of tubulinopathies: what are the key features for the diagnosis? *Brain* **2014**, *137*, 1676–1700. [CrossRef] [PubMed]
7. Sanders, S.J.; Murtha, M.T.; Gupta, A.R.; Murdoch, J.D.; Raubeson, M.J.; Willsey, A.J.; Ercan-Sencicek, A.G.; DiLullo, N.M.; Parikshak, N.N.; Stein, J.L.; et al. De novo mutations revealed by whole-exome sequencing are strongly associated with autism. *Nature* **2012**, *485*, 237–241. [CrossRef] [PubMed]
8. McMichael, G.; Girirajan, S.; Moreno-De-Luca, A.; Gecz, J.; Shard, C.; Nguyen, L.S.; Nicholl, J.; Gibson, C.; Haan, E.; Eichler, E.; et al. Rare copy number variation in cerebral palsy. *Eur. J. Hum. Genet.* **2014**, *22*, 40–45. [CrossRef] [PubMed]
9. Yokoi, S.; Ishihara, N.; Miya, F.; Tsutsumi, M.; Yanagihara, I.; Fujita, N.; Yamamoto, H.; Kato, M.; Okamoto, N.; Tsunoda, T.; et al. TUBA1A mutation can cause a hydranencephaly-like severe form of cortical dysgenesis. *Sci. Rep.* **2015**, *5*, 15165. [CrossRef] [PubMed]
10. Jaglin, X.H.; Poirier, K.; Saillour, Y.; Buhler, E.; Tian, G.; Bahi-Buisson, N.; Fallet-Bianco, C.; Phan-Dinh-Tuy, F.; Kong, X.P.; Bomont, P.; et al. Mutations in the beta-tubulin gene *TUBB2B* result in asymmetrical polymicrogyria. *Nat. Genet.* **2009**, *41*, 746–752. [CrossRef] [PubMed]
11. Tischfield, M.A.; Baris, H.N.; Wu, C.; Rudolph, G.; Van Maldergem, L.; He, W.; Chan, W.-M.; Andrews, C.; Demer, J.L.; Robertson, R.L.; et al. Human TUBB3 mutations perturb microtubule dynamics, kinesin interactions, and axon guidance. *Cell* **2010**, *140*, 74–87. [CrossRef] [PubMed]
12. Poirier, K.; Saillour, Y.; Bahi-Buisson, N.; Jaglin, X.H.; Fallet-Bianco, C.; Nabbout, R.; Castelnau-Ptakhine, L.; Roubertie, A.; Attie-Bitach, T.; Desguerre, I.; et al. Mutations in the neuronal β-tubulin subunit TUBB3 result in malformation of cortical development and neuronal migration defects. *Hum. Mol. Genet.* **2010**, *19*, 4462–4473. [CrossRef] [PubMed]
13. Breuss, M.; Heng, J.I.-T.; Poirier, K.; Tian, G.; Jaglin, X.H.; Qu, Z.; Braun, A.; Gstrein, T.; Ngo, L.; Haas, M.; et al. Mutations in the β-tubulin gene *TUBB5* cause microcephaly with structural brain abnormalities. *Cell Rep.* **2012**, *2*, 1554–1562. [CrossRef] [PubMed]
14. Cushion, T.D.; Paciorkowski, A.R.; Pilz, D.T.; Mullins, J.G.L.; Seltzer, L.E.; Marion, R.W.; Tuttle, E.; Ghoneim, D.; Christian, S.L.; Chung, S.-K.; et al. De novo mutations in the beta-tubulin gene *TUBB2A* cause simplified gyral patterning and infantile-onset epilepsy. *Am. J. Hum. Genet.* **2014**, *94*, 634–641. [CrossRef] [PubMed]
15. Poirier, K.; Lebrun, N.; Broix, L.; Tian, G.; Saillour, Y.; Boscheron, C.; Parrini, E.; Valence, S.; Pierre, B.S.; Oger, M.; et al. Mutations in TUBG1, DYNC1H1, KIF5C and KIF2A cause malformations of cortical development and microcephaly. *Nat. Genet.* **2013**, *45*, 639–647. [CrossRef] [PubMed]
16. Romaniello, R.; Arrigoni, F.; Panzeri, E.; Poretti, A.; Micalizzi, A.; Citterio, A.; Bedeschi, M.F.; Berardinelli, A.; Cusmai, R.; D'Arrigo, S.; et al. Tubulin-related cerebellar dysplasia: definition of a distinct pattern of cerebellar malformation. *Eur. Radiol.* **2017**, *27*, 5080–5092. [CrossRef] [PubMed]
17. Kumar, R.A.; Pilz, D.T.; Babatz, T.D.; Cushion, T.D.; Harvey, K.; Topf, M.; Yates, L.; Robb, S.; Uyanik, G.; Mancini, G.M.S.; et al. TUBA1A mutations cause wide spectrum lissencephaly (smooth brain) and suggest that multiple neuronal migration pathways converge on alpha tubulins. *Hum. Mol. Genet.* **2010**, *19*, 2817–2827. [CrossRef] [PubMed]
18. Bahi-Buisson, N.; Poirier, K.; Boddaert, N.; Saillour, Y.; Castelnau, L.; Philip, N.; Buyse, G.; Villard, L.; Joriot, S.; Marret, S.; et al. Refinement of cortical dysgeneses spectrum associated with TUBA1A mutations. *J. Med. Genet.* **2008**, *45*, 647–653. [CrossRef] [PubMed]
19. Poirier, K.; Keays, D.A.; Francis, F.; Saillour, Y.; Bahi, N.; Manouvrier, S.; Fallet-Bianco, C.; Pasquier, L.; Toutain, A.; Tuy, F.P.D.; et al. Large spectrum of lissencephaly and pachygyria phenotypes resulting from de novo missense mutations in tubulin alpha 1A (TUBA1A). *Hum. Mutat.* **2007**, *28*, 1055–1064. [CrossRef] [PubMed]

20. Tian, G.; Kong, X.-P.; Jaglin, X.H.; Chelly, J.; Keays, D.; Cowan, N.J. A pachygyria-causing alpha-tubulin mutation results in inefficient cycling with CCT and a deficient interaction with TBCB. *Mol. Biol. Cell* **2008**, *19*, 1152–1161. [CrossRef] [PubMed]
21. Farwell, K.D.; Shahmirzadi, L.; El-Khechen, D.; Powis, Z.; Chao, E.C.; Tippin Davis, B.; Baxter, R.M.; Zeng, W.; Mroske, C.; Parra, M.C.; et al. Enhanced utility of family-centered diagnostic exome sequencing with inheritance model-based analysis: results from 500 unselected families with undiagnosed genetic conditions. *Genet. Med.* **2015**, *17*, 578–586. [CrossRef] [PubMed]
22. Alby, C.; Malan, V.; Boutaud, L.; Marangoni, M.A.; Bessières, B.; Bonniere, M.; Ichkou, A.; Elkhartoufi, N.; Bahi-Buisson, N.; Sonigo, P.; et al. Clinical, genetic and neuropathological findings in a series of 138 fetuses with a corpus callosum malformation. *Birth Defects Res. Part A Clin. Mol. Teratol.* **2016**, *106*, 36–46. [CrossRef] [PubMed]
23. Srivastava, S.; Cohen, J.S.; Vernon, H.; Barañano, K.; McClellan, R.; Jamal, L.; Naidu, S.; Fatemi, A. Clinical whole exome sequencing in child neurology practice. *Ann. Neurol.* **2014**, *76*, 473–483. [CrossRef] [PubMed]
24. Alby, C.; Boutaud, L.; Bessières, B.; Serre, V.; Rio, M.; Cormier-Daire, V.; de Oliveira, J.; Ichkou, A.; Mouthon, L.; Gordon, C.T.; et al. Novel de novo ZBTB20 mutations in three cases with Primrose syndrome and constant corpus callosum anomalies. *Am. J. Med. Genet. A* **2018**, *176*, 1091–1098. [CrossRef] [PubMed]
25. Alby, C.; Boutaud, L.; Bonnière, M.; Collardeau-Frachon, S.; Guibaud, L.; Lopez, E.; Bruel, A.-L.; Aral, B.; Sonigo, P.; Roth, P.; et al. In utero ultrasound diagnosis of corpus callosum agenesis leading to the identification of orofaciodigital type 1 syndrome in female fetuses. *Birth Defects Res.* **2018**, *110*, 382–389. [CrossRef] [PubMed]
26. Mullins, J.G.L. Structural modelling pipelines in next generation sequencing projects. *Adv. Protein Chem. Struct. Biol.* **2012**, *89*, 117–167. [CrossRef] [PubMed]
27. Prota, A.E.; Bargsten, K.; Zurwerra, D.; Field, J.J.; Díaz, J.F.; Altmann, K.-H.; Steinmetz, M.O. Molecular mechanism of action of microtubule-stabilizing anticancer agents. *Science* **2013**, *339*, 587–590. [CrossRef] [PubMed]
28. Fourniol, F.J.; Sindelar, C.V.; Amigues, B.; Clare, D.K.; Thomas, G.; Perderiset, M.; Francis, F.; Houdusse, A.; Moores, C.A. Template-free 13-protofilament microtubule-MAP assembly visualized at 8 A resolution. *J. Cell Biol.* **2010**, *191*, 463–470. [CrossRef] [PubMed]
29. Webb, B.; Sali, A. Comparative Protein Structure Modeling Using MODELLER. *Curr. Protoc. Bioinform.* **2016**, *54*, 5.6.1–5.6.37. [CrossRef]
30. Pettersen, E.F.; Goddard, T.D.; Huang, C.C.; Couch, G.S.; Greenblatt, D.M.; Meng, E.C.; Ferrin, T.E. UCSF Chimera—A visualization system for exploratory research and analysis. *J. Comput. Chem.* **2004**, *25*, 1605–1612. [CrossRef] [PubMed]
31. UCSF Chimera Home Page. Available online: https://www.cgl.ucsf.edu/chimera/ (accessed on 23 July 2018).
32. Ensembl Genome Browser 93. Available online: http://www.ensembl.org/index.html (accessed on 23 July 2018).
33. Aggarwala, V.; Voight, B.F. An expanded sequence context model broadly explains variability in polymorphism levels across the human genome. *Nat. Genet.* **2016**, *48*, 349–355. [CrossRef] [PubMed]
34. Wildeman, M.; van Ophuizen, E.; den Dunnen, J.T.; Taschner, P.E.M. Improving sequence variant descriptions in mutation databases and literature using the Mutalyzer sequence variation nomenclature checker. *Hum. Mutat.* **2008**, *29*, 6–13. [CrossRef] [PubMed]
35. Mutalyzer 2.0.28—Welcome to the Mutalyzer Website. Available online: https://www.mutalyzer.nl/ (accessed on 23 July 2018).
36. Oegema, R.; Cushion, T.D.; Phelps, I.G.; Chung, S.-K.; Dempsey, J.C.; Collins, S.; Mullins, J.G.L.; Dudding, T.; Gill, H.; Green, A.J.; et al. Recognizable cerebellar dysplasia associated with mutations in multiple tubulin genes. *Hum. Mol. Genet.* **2015**, *24*, 5313–5325. [CrossRef] [PubMed]
37. Poirier, K.; Saillour, Y.; Fourniol, F.; Francis, F.; Souville, I.; Valence, S.; Desguerre, I.; Marie Lepage, J.; Boddaert, N.; Line Jacquemont, M.; et al. Expanding the spectrum of TUBA1A-related cortical dysgenesis to Polymicrogyria. *Eur. J. Hum. Genet.* **2013**, *21*, 381–385. [CrossRef] [PubMed]
38. Kamiya, K.; Tanaka, F.; Ikeno, M.; Okumura, A.; Aoki, S. DTI tractography of lissencephaly caused by *TUBA1A* mutation. *Neurol. Sci.* **2014**, *35*, 801–803. [CrossRef] [PubMed]
39. Mokánszki, A.; Körhegyi, I.; Szabó, N.; Bereg, E.; Gergev, G.; Balogh, E.; Bessenyei, B.; Sümegi, A.; Morris-Rosendahl, D.J.; Sztriha, L.; et al. Lissencephaly and band heterotopia: LIS1, TUBA1A, and DCX mutations in Hungary. *J. Child Neurol.* **2012**, *27*, 1534–1540. [CrossRef] [PubMed]

40. Morris-Rosendahl, D.J.; Najm, J.; Lachmeijer, A.M.A.; Sztriha, L.; Martins, M.; Kuechler, A.; Haug, V.; Zeschnigk, C.; Martin, P.; Santos, M.; et al. Refining the phenotype of alpha-1a Tubulin (TUBA1A) mutation in patients with classical lissencephaly. *Clin. Genet.* **2008**, *74*, 425–433. [CrossRef] [PubMed]
41. Feng, R.; Sang, Q.; Kuang, Y.; Sun, X.; Yan, Z.; Zhang, S.; Shi, J.; Tian, G.; Luchniak, A.; Fukuda, Y.; et al. Mutations in TUBB8 and Human Oocyte Meiotic Arrest. *N. Engl. J. Med.* **2016**, *374*, 223–232. [CrossRef] [PubMed]
42. Chen, B.; Li, B.; Li, D.; Yan, Z.; Mao, X.; Xu, Y.; Mu, J.; Li, Q.; Jin, L.; He, L.; et al. Novel mutations and structural deletions in *TUBB8*: Expanding mutational and phenotypic spectrum of patients with arrest in oocyte maturation, fertilization or early embryonic development. *Hum. Reprod.* **2017**, *32*, 457–464. [CrossRef] [PubMed]
43. Huang, L.; Tong, X.; Luo, L.; Zheng, S.; Jin, R.; Fu, Y.; Zhou, G.; Li, D.; Liu, Y. Mutation analysis of the *TUBB8* gene in nine infertile women with oocyte maturation arrest. *Reprod. Biomed. Online* **2017**, *35*, 305–310. [CrossRef] [PubMed]
44. Lohmann, K.; Wilcox, R.A.; Winkler, S.; Ramirez, A.; Rakovic, A.; Park, J.-S.; Arns, B.; Lohnau, T.; Groen, J.; Kasten, M.; et al. Whispering dysphonia (DYT4 dystonia) is caused by a mutation in the *TUBB4* gene. *Ann. Neurol.* **2013**, *73*, 537–545. [CrossRef] [PubMed]
45. Hersheson, J.; Mencacci, N.E.; Davis, M.; MacDonald, N.; Trabzuni, D.; Ryten, M.; Pittman, A.; Paudel, R.; Kara, E.; Fawcett, K.; et al. Mutations in the autoregulatory domain of β-tubulin 4a cause hereditary dystonia. *Ann. Neurol.* **2013**, *73*, 546–553. [CrossRef] [PubMed]
46. Hamilton, E.M.; Polder, E.; Vanderver, A.; Naidu, S.; Schiffmann, R.; Fisher, K.; Raguž, A.B.; Blumkin, L.; H-ABC Research Group; van Berkel, C.G.M.; et al. Hypomyelination with atrophy of the basal ganglia and cerebellum: further delineation of the phenotype and genotype-phenotype correlation. *Brain* **2014**, *137*, 1921–1930. [CrossRef] [PubMed]
47. Miyatake, S.; Osaka, H.; Shiina, M.; Sasaki, M.; Takanashi, J.-I.; Haginoya, K.; Wada, T.; Morimoto, M.; Ando, N.; Ikuta, Y.; et al. Expanding the phenotypic spectrum of TUBB4A-associated hypomyelinating leukoencephalopathies. *Neurology* **2014**, *82*, 2230–2237. [CrossRef] [PubMed]
48. Simons, C.; Wolf, N.I.; McNeil, N.; Caldovic, L.; Devaney, J.M.; Takanohashi, A.; Crawford, J.; Ru, K.; Grimmond, S.M.; Miller, D.; et al. A de novo mutation in the β-tubulin gene *TUBB4A* results in the leukoencephalopathy hypomyelination with atrophy of the basal ganglia and cerebellum. *Am. J. Hum. Genet.* **2013**, *92*, 767–773. [CrossRef] [PubMed]

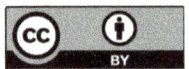

© 2018 by the authors. Licensee MDPI, Basel, Switzerland. This article is an open access article distributed under the terms and conditions of the Creative Commons Attribution (CC BY) license (http://creativecommons.org/licenses/by/4.0/).

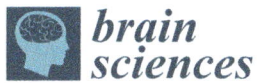

Review

The Role of Movement Analysis in Diagnosing and Monitoring Neurodegenerative Conditions: Insights from Gait and Postural Control

Christopher Buckley [1,†], Lisa Alcock [1,†], Ríona McArdle [1], Rana Zia Ur Rehman [1], Silvia Del Din [1], Claudia Mazzà [2], Alison J. Yarnall [1,3] and Lynn Rochester [1,3,*]

1. Institute of Neuroscience/Institute for Ageing, Newcastle University, Newcastle Upon Tyne NE4 5PL, UK; christopher.buckley2@newcastle.ac.uk (C.B.); Lisa.Alcock@newcastle.ac.uk (L.A.); R.Mc-Ardle2@newcastle.ac.uk (R.M.); Rana.zia-ur-Rehman@newcastle.ac.uk (R.Z.U.R.); Silvia.Del-Din@newcastle.ac.uk (S.D.D.); alison.yarnall@newcastle.ac.uk (A.J.Y.)
2. Department of Mechanical Engineering, Sheffield University, Sheffield S1 3JD, UK; c.mazza@sheffield.ac.uk
3. The Newcastle upon Tyne Hospitals NHS Foundation Trust, Newcastle Upon Tyne NE7 7DN, UK
* Correspondence: lynn.rochester@ncl.ac.uk; Tel.: +0191-208-1291 (direct line); +44-191-208-1250 (reception); Fax: +44-191-208-1251
† These authors contributed equally.

Received: 18 January 2019; Accepted: 31 January 2019; Published: 6 February 2019

Abstract: Quantifying gait and postural control adds valuable information that aids in understanding neurological conditions where motor symptoms predominate and cause considerable functional impairment. Disease-specific clinical scales exist; however, they are often susceptible to subjectivity, and can lack sensitivity when identifying subtle gait and postural impairments in prodromal cohorts and longitudinally to document disease progression. Numerous devices are available to objectively quantify a range of measurement outcomes pertaining to gait and postural control; however, efforts are required to standardise and harmonise approaches that are specific to the neurological condition and clinical assessment. Tools are urgently needed that address a number of unmet needs in neurological practice. Namely, these include timely and accurate diagnosis; disease stratification; risk prediction; tracking disease progression; and decision making for intervention optimisation and maximising therapeutic response (such as medication selection, disease staging, and targeted support). Using some recent examples of research across a range of relevant neurological conditions—including Parkinson's disease, ataxia, and dementia—we will illustrate evidence that supports progress against these unmet clinical needs. We summarise the novel 'big data' approaches that utilise data mining and machine learning techniques to improve disease classification and risk prediction, and conclude with recommendations for future direction.

Keywords: movement science; Parkinson's disease; ataxia; dementia; machine learning; deep learning; risk prediction; disease phenotyping

1. Introduction

Quantifying movement through clinical observation is central to enhancing our understanding of neurological disorders. It informs diagnosis, disease severity, progression, and therapeutic response. Mobility deficits (particularly gait and postural control, which form the focus of this review) provide critical information relevant to the diagnostic process. The clinical assessment of gait and posture within an outpatient, inpatient, or rehabilitation setting typically takes the form of self-report, subjective scales, and observation. Validated gait and postural control rating scales and assessments are also commonly applied (e.g., the Tinetti Performance-Oriented Mobility Assessment [1], the Dynamic Gait Index [2], and the Berg Balance Scale [3,4]). Although helpful in terms of change over time and considered the gold standard in clinical settings, significant limitations exist, due to variation, subjectivity, inconsistency, and poor granularity. Moreover, as we move to an era where the focus is on earlier detection, different tools are needed with greater sensitivity to detect change than is currently offered.

Traditional approaches to quantify gait and postural control have relied upon complex and expensive laboratory equipment and specialist expertise, which lack translation to the clinic. Developments in movement analysis devices such as reduced prices and improved automated software are now facilitating their applicability not only to clinics but also for continuous monitoring on a large scale within real-world settings. The opportunity for better protocol standardisation, the harmonisation of outcome measures, and assessments of large cohorts through multi-centre studies in this evolving field are a welcome consequence. Equally welcome is the opportunity for improved stratification for clinical trials of novel neuroprotective therapies and disease progression. In an era of personalised medicine and early detection of risk, subtle changes in movement consequent to neurodegenerative disease would also improve clinical management through timely and accurate diagnosis and tracking, disease stratification, risk prediction, and enhanced decision making for intervention optimisation and maximising therapeutic response (such as medication selection, disease staging, and targeted support). In turn, the improved information provided with the correct interpretation may improve independence, quality of life, and a reduction of fall risk for patients.

Throughout this review of the scientific literature, we will focus on the role of quantitative movement analysis in neurodegenerative disorders and restrict our discussion to the measurement of gait and postural control measured during standing in key conditions. The review has four sections, each of which addresses a key aim. Section I aims to provide an overview of the strengths and limitations of current measurement techniques/devices, outcomes, and protocols relevant to key measurement needs. Section II aims to provide evidence to support the use of gait and postural control as clinical biomarkers as defined above, drawing from studies in Parkinson's disease (PD), ataxia, and dementia. Section III aims to highlight new and emerging areas relating to bioinformatics (data mining and machine learning) and what we can learn in the context of disease classification, phenotyping, and risk prediction. Finally, Section IV offers recommendations for future work in this field.

2. Section I: Quantitative Movement Analysis: From Measurement Tools to Outcome Measures

Below, we provide a brief overview of the measurement tools, protocols, and quantitative outcome measures that are currently utilised, highlighting the most relevant (Figure 1 and Table 1).

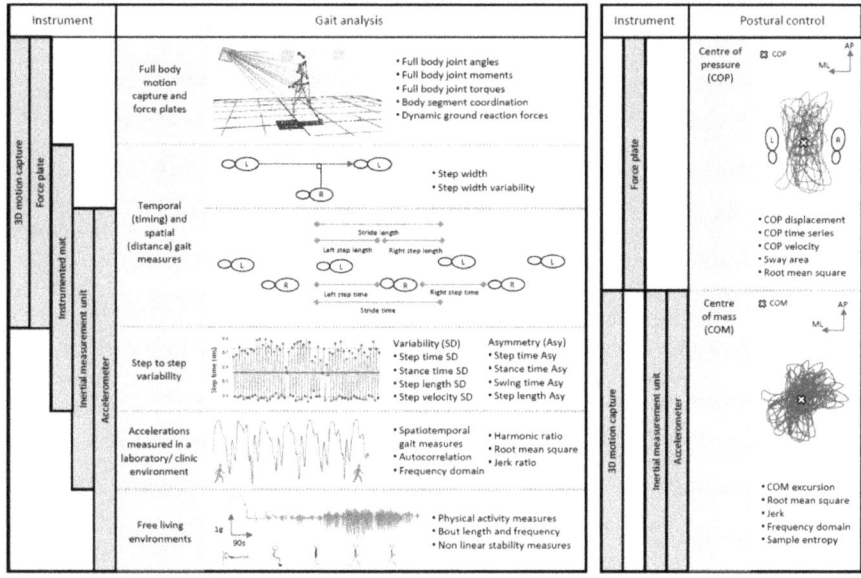

Figure 1. Summary of outcome measures that may be obtained from a quantitative assessment of gait and postural control.

Table 1. A summary of the advantages and disadvantages of measurement devices used to quantify gait and postural control. COP: center of pressure.

Device	Advantages	Disadvantages
3D motion capture	- Considered the gold standard - Highly precise and accurate - Potential to measure a large variety of outcomes - Non-invasive - High-resolution data	- High cost - Requires experienced technical expertise - Requires a large purpose-built dedicated space usually limited to laboratory/research environments - Participant preparation can be time-consuming
Force plates	- Considered gold standard for measuring ground reaction forces and COP - Non-invasive - Minimal space required - Minimal participant preparation time - High-resolution data	- High cost - Requires experienced technical expertise - Requires a purpose-built dedicated space
Instrumented mats	- Minimal processing time - Non-invasive - Minimal participant preparation time - Portable	- Extractable features are limited by mat dimensions - Requires a large space to accommodate the mat dimensions - Limited to temporal spatial and foot pressure gait outcomes of the lower extremities
Inertial measurement units	- Capable of capturing continuous movements in laboratory and community environments - Non-invasive with minimal participant preparation time - Certain systems provide automated reports - Cheaper than the gold standard - Portable	- Often requires complex algorithms and special expertise to extract key features - Features are often indirect measures requiring additional participant measurements - Free-living measurements may be limited by recording time (if battery powered) or data storage (if data is stored internally on the device)
Accelerometer	- Low cost - Wearable, wireless technology capable of capturing continuous movements in lab and community environments for prolonged periods (>one week) - Non-invasive - Minimal participant preparation time - Portable	- Often requires complex algorithms and special expertise to extract key features post-data collection - Features are often indirect measures requiring additional participant measurements - Data collected in community living environments lack context

2.1. Quantifying Gait and Postural Control—Which Tools?

For an objective, quantitative analysis of gait and postural control, three-dimensional motion analysis, footswitches, instrumented walkways, body-worn sensors, pressure mats, force platforms, posturography, and electromyography are the most common tools, each with their own strengths and limitations. Quantitative tools can be as simple as a stopwatch, which with a known distance, can be used to gain clinically relevant measures such as gait speed [5]. The main consideration when deciding the best approach is the need to balance the requirement for better granularity, sensitivity, specificity, measurement accuracy, and minimal rater bias, with the complexity and feasibility of using such methods in clinics, communities, and clinical trials (Table 1).

Three-dimensional motion analysis systems are capable of measuring movements of the whole body; they can measure both gait and postural control, are highly accurate and precise, and are relied upon as the gold standard to compare new tools as well as to evaluate the benefit of therapeutic interventions (e.g., surgical procedures, pharmacological therapies, assistive devices, and exercise training programs) [6]. However, the high cost, long preparation time, and need for specialist staff to operate these systems are barriers to their wholesale adoption within routine clinical care [7]. Furthermore, even when clinically implemented, the choices regarding protocols such as different marker sets and biomechanical models, which are needed to quantify kinetics and kinematics, combined with the complexity of the outputs, can greatly influence the outcome and decisions based on the data collected [8]. This means that these systems are largely limited to research settings.

Instrumented mats provide reliable quantitative spatiotemporal gait characteristics of the feet at a lower cost relative to three-dimensional motion analysis, while also providing pressure information [9–11]. They can provide a number of gait outcomes ranging from information on pace to dynamic postural control [12]. If located in a dedicated space, the preparation time for the device and the participant is minimal. Additionally, most systems come packaged with accompanying software that is capable of generating automated reports, meaning that specialist support may not always be required. Limitations include: the devices are not easily portable and require large indoor spaces, are not capable of measuring standing balance, and that due to the finite size of the mat, multiple trials are required to generate reliable gait measures [13].

More recently, technological advances in wearable devices allow an alternative to traditional laboratory-based and clinical assessments of gait and postural control. Wearable sensors are mobile devices that are designed to be worn on the body, or embedded into watches, bracelets, and clothing [14]. They may be used in the clinic, but also in free living. This opens a whole new perspective in terms of assessing mobility over extended periods of time [15–18] while concurrently evaluating traditional and novel measures of gait [19,20], quantitative measures of physical activity [21], and postural outcomes such as transitions and turns [22,23]. The inclusion of free-living data alone or in addition to clinical assessment provides vital information that may help inform the diagnosis and monitoring of neurological disease. However, whilst these new avenues and variables appear promising, the best combination of methods and metrics are still to be determined [15,24]. However, limitations with wearable devices should be considered. Although a single accelerometer is inexpensive relative to the other more traditional devices highlighted above, multiple sensor systems with accompanying software that is capable of calculating outcome measures into reports dramatically increase the price. Also, with such systems, clinicians require methodological training, which is critical for avoiding blind interpretations of erroneous reports. Lastly, although many proxy measures of gait have been validated [25,26], many algorithms for their estimate and novel measures have not, meaning that further effort is needed in order to create robust, validated, and population-specific normative values.

2.2. Outcome Measures and Data Collection Protocols

Below, we provide a brief summary of some of the most common outcomes from quantitative analysis that are used to describe gait and postural control (Figure 1). Gait and postural control are intimately related. Gait models include measures that reflect aspects of gait-related postural control, and can be interpreted as such. However, for the purposes of this review and to reflect how assessment is commonly conducted, we address each independently.

For gait, the most common outcome is gait speed because of its robust clinimetric properties [5,12]. Often regarded as a global measure of overall function, gait speed is informative; however, it does not reveal the specific gait deficit (i.e., temporal or spatial control of gait), and as such is limited [12]. Moreover, in laboratory and clinical settings, gait speed may also be susceptible to the 'Hawthorne effect', whereby participants perform particularly well in controlled environments whilst being observed [27]. Many other outcomes can be used to describe gait, and may add greater specificity regarding differentiating between neurological conditions and increased sensitivity when evaluating subtle within-person changes [12,28]. To aid interpretation, normative values have been published and serve as reference data [29,30], and conceptual models of gait have been developed to provide a more structured approach [12,31,32].

The measurement of gait can be broadly grouped within a structure that captures: (1) spatiotemporal features that reflect a typical gait cycle, which is expressed as the average of multiple steps over a specified distance; and (2) dynamic features of gait, which represent the step-by-step inconsistency of spatiotemporal measures across these steps [12]. These dynamic features are typically represented by the within-person standard deviation (SD) or the coefficient of variation [33]. Hausdorff (2009) [34] also introduced a broader definition of the dynamic features of gait that incorporated the underlying structure and pattern of movements in gait derived from data collected over longer periods. These long-term, fractal-like correlations break down with age and disease, and as such, different measures reflecting the variability of movement may provide additional sensitive markers of early/prodromal disease [34].

Standardised protocols for the assessment of gait (for a recent review, see [35]) typically measure gait at a preferred walking speed over four metres, and are clinically applicable [36]. Departure from this protocol is acceptable for some gait characteristics, but not for others. Gait speed is reliable over 10 m or six minutes, for both preferred and fast walking, and in clinic and home environments [26,37–40]. This is not the case for gait variability, where clinimetrics improve with a greater number of steps, and a minimum of 30 steps is advocated [13,41,42]. Walking over longer durations (e.g., two and six-minute walking tests) are also commonly used to infer endurance [43]. Protocols are also modified to provide additional challenge; these are so-called "stress tests". They include dual-task paradigms, turning, backward walking, and walking at a fast pace [44]. Dual-task testing paradigms (i.e., asking someone to recall a sequence of numbers while walking) are employed to reduce the compensatory cognitive control of gait, revealing latent motor deficits; as a consequence, they also expose the level of compensatory cognitive control that is required to maintain gait performance.

A range of outcomes exist for measuring postural control during standing. Typically, they are derived from either movements of the center of mass (COM) or the center of pressure (COP), and can be summarised as linear and non-linear outcomes (see Figure 1). Linear parameters and derived indexes provide information about the direction (e.g., anterior–posterior or mediolateral directions) and global 'magnitude' of postural sway (e.g., root mean square (RMS), limits of stability, jerk, ellipsis), and the fluctuation of COM or COP displacement (frequency domain metrics) [45–52]. Non-linear outcomes describe the regularity or predictability of balance control [53].

The protocols that are used to assess postural control vary greatly from quiet standing to standing barefoot or with shoes on, on a foam support or firm surface, with eyes open or closed (Romberg test), with either standardised or unrestricted foot placement, with arms across the chest or by their sides, and over different trial durations ranging from 30 to 120 seconds [48,51,53–56]. To date, postural control outcomes are typically summarised over the test duration, which may limit comparability across protocols of varied duration, as most linear metrics are time-dependent and thus influenced by test duration. For example, a person's total COM excursion will increase relative to time, highlighting the need for normalisation and standardised protocols for between-investigation comparisons (for a detailed description of how method can impact postural control measures, please see [57]). Alterations in postural control over discrete windows of time may provide a more subtle reflection of postural adaptations in addition to outcomes averaged across the test duration [56].

In summary, the breadth of tools that are used to measure gait and postural control are vast, as are the range of protocols for data collection and the outcome measures that are extracted. Therefore, there is a need to standardise and harmonise approaches. Currently, the optimal testing battery for gait and postural control applied either independently or in combination is unknown, and further work is needed to define this on a disease-by-disease basis, and also with respect to the purpose (e.g., diagnosis, progression, risk prediction), as one size will not fit all. The opportunity for the uncontrolled continuous monitoring of gait and postural control during free-living activities is an area of considerable interest, and its additional measurement holds promise for the future. A growing number of outcomes may be obtained ranging from the micro (i.e., step length and time) to the macro (i.e., total time walking per day) features of gait. However, the optimal approach to integrate free-living movements into clinical decision making is yet to be defined, and this continues to be an area of emerging interest. Despite this, the promise of movement analysis for diagnosing and monitoring neurological conditions is becoming increasingly evident, and examples from recent literature are highlighted in Section II across a range of different disease groups.

3. Section II: Distinguishing Features of Gait and Postural Control across Neurodegenerative Conditions

In this section, we highlight examples from the recent literature to illustrate the value of instrumented assessment of gait and postural control across a range of different disease groups.

3.1. Parkinson's Disease

Parkinson's disease (PD) is the second most common neurodegenerative disease after Alzheimer's disease (AD), affecting one in every 500 adults in the United Kingdom (UK) and up to 10 million worldwide [58–60]. PD was previously described as a degeneration of dopaminergic cells in the substantia nigra; however, a more contemporary understanding of PD highlights that it is a complex multi-system disorder that is represented clinically by a syndrome with multiple neurotransmitter deficits (for a recent review, see [61]). A variety of clinical assessment scales have been designed to evaluate the motor symptoms of PD (including gait and postural control) such as the Unified Parkinson's disease rating scale Part 3 (UPDRSIII [62]) and the Hoehn and Yahr scale [63]. They are embedded within routine clinical evaluation and categorically grade disease severity and motor symptoms from normal to severe. As such, they often do not capture detailed information regarding motor deficits, may miss subtle within-person changes, and can be susceptible to variation when administered by different assessors.

The quantification of gait characteristics in PD can inform risk [64], progression (including response to treatment) [65], and diagnosis [66]. Notably, discrete gait changes predict both future falls [67,68] and cognitive decline in incident PD [69], raising the possibility of a target for a preventative approach in early disease. Subtle and discrete differences have been identified in early PD compared to age-matched controls, with reduced step length, increased asymmetry, and step-to-step variability [65]. Gait impairments evolve over time from a subtle, discrete picture to a more global presentation of deficit in all its characteristics [65,70,71]. Subtle gait impairments are also present in individuals with Parkinson's 'at risk' syndromes such as rapid eye movement (REM) and sleep behavior disorder (RBD) prior to the development of Parkinsonian features (so-called 'prodromal' disease) when compared to healthy controls without risk factors [72].

Monitoring upper-body movements (such as the magnitude of arm swing or movement of the trunk) during walking is emerging as a powerful measure complementary to traditional gait analysis (measuring stepping characteristics), and has been shown to be capable of discriminating PD from controls [24,73], and PD fallers from non-fallers [74–76]. Arm swing variability during gait has also been identified as a distinguishing feature in carriers of the G2019S mutation, which was significantly different to both non-carriers and people with PD [77]. This has raised the possibility of upper body movements during gait as a clinical biomarker for PD to enhance diagnostic accuracy, which in early disease may only be between 70–80% [78], and supports the use of quantitative, objective assessments to measure changes that may not be detected during routine clinical observation.

Gait continues to deteriorate even in the early stages of the disease despite optimal medication with evidence to suggest that some discrete characteristics of gait are dopa-resistant (i.e., step length, step width, and swing time) [65,71]. Other gait characteristics appear to be responsive to intervention, with a recent review of pharmacological therapies highlighting the role of cholinesterase inhibitors to improve gait variability [79]. Therefore, quantitative movement analysis may be useful when understanding the effectiveness of levodopa, and potentially highlight when alternative treatment options may be required. Deficits in gait have been linked to primary pathophysiology, as visualised with functional and structural neuroimaging, cerebral spinal fluid, and blood-based biomarkers, supporting the use of discrete gait characteristics as potential clinical biomarkers to track pathology. Gait impairments such as gait speed may be attributed to underlying cholinergic dysfunction [80,81], with evidence to suggest that amyloid proteinopathies may also contribute to the progression of dopa-resistant gait characteristics (step time and length variability) [71]. Freezing of gait (FOG) is a debilitating symptom that often affects patients with advanced PD, and has shown a positive response to levodopa [67]. FOG is recognised as an episodic absence or marked reduction of forward progression of the feet, despite the intention to walk [82], and is associated with an impaired regulation of stride variability [83–86]. A recent report explored the potential use of smartphones to assess digital biomarkers of PD, including gait and postural control, and to identify exploratory outcome measures for Phase I clinical trials [87]. The results revealed acceptable adherence and moderate to strong retest reliability (Intraclass Correlation Coefficient = 0.84), highlighting the potential of using smartphones to collect gait and postural control data. Not only were people with PD distinguished successfully from controls, the analysis of turning (possible with accelerometer and gyroscope-derived measures) offered increased sensitivity compared to traditional clinical scales [87].

Previous research quantifying the linear parameters of postural control has suggested that: (i) abnormalities in postural control during quiet standing exist even in early PD [45,46,56]; (ii) linear parameters can differentiate between PD motor subtypes [88]; and (iii) as disease symptoms progress, sway parameters deteriorate, especially in the mediolateral direction [45]. The positive effect of dopaminergic replacement therapy that has been observed for gait may not be paralleled for postural control, where levodopa has been shown to worsen some outcomes [50]. Non-linear measures of postural control have shown that people with PD display lower predictability/regularity of the COM along all sway directions; this may be explained by the loss of constant fine adjustments of posture due to impaired sensorimotor integration and the disturbance of habitual motor control pathways [53]. However, it is still unclear whether regularity metrics are sensitive to disease progression [53,89]. However, practically, monitoring the positive and negative influence of therapies may be useful in clinical management and falls risk.

3.2. Ataxia

The prevalence of hereditary cerebellar ataxias is estimated at 2.7/100,000 (average derived from meta-analyses [90]). Ataxia describes a collection of neurological disorders affecting the cerebellum that impair the control and coordination of whole body movements, eye movements (nystagmus), and speech (dysarthria) [44,91,92]. Consequently, the integration of sensory information to coordinate voluntary movements is challenged, and impairs gait and postural control. Poor gait control is often the initial symptom in ataxia groups [93], reportedly occurring in around 60% of ataxia patients [94], and in some cases emerging prior to the onset of neurological symptoms [95]. Quantitative movement analysis has shown that ataxic gait is associated with slower walking speeds and a reduced cadence, a shorter step and swing phase duration, a longer double limb support phase, wider steps, and increased gait variability (particularly step length and width) [96–104]. Impaired gait and postural control are associated with an increased falls risk [99,105,106], and serve as attractive targets for intervention (refer to [107,108] for comprehensive reviews of gait and balance, respectively). Falls are common in people with ataxia, occurring in up to 74%, and prevalence is proportionate to other neurological conditions such as PD [109]. We draw upon examples of inherited and secondary ataxias [110,111] to highlight the importance of quantitative analysis of gait and postural control in this patient group. While broad clinical scales such as the Scale for the Assessment and Rating of Ataxia (SARA) [112] provide an indication of overall function, they are unable to reveal the nature of subtle movement impairments in this patient group. Quantifiable, objective measures that may be used as markers to document gait and postural impairment are lacking when relying on these clinical scales alone. Gait variability, in particular variability in the timing of movement, is specific to cerebellar dysfunction [113], and cannot be assessed using clinical scales.

Patients with ataxic symptoms, including individuals with multiple sclerosis, display deficits in postural control including a greater magnitude and speed of postural sway [97,114], which is attributed to a reduced range of motion at the knee ('locked knees') and a delayed response in muscle activity [115]. To compensate for this poor postural control, people with ataxia often widen their stance (base of support) to stabilise the head and trunk [116]. Anterior–posterior falls are more common than falls in the mediolateral direction [117]. Accordingly, assessment protocols that assess balance in the anterior–posterior direction pose a heightened challenge for people with ataxia [118,119].

Quantifiable measurement outcomes obtained during gait are useful for distinguishing ataxia and mitochondrial disease from controls and other neurological conditions such as PD and hereditary spastic paraplegia (HSP) [100,120,121]. For example, patients with mitochondrial disease walk slower, with a shorter step and increased step width variability during normal and dual task walking compared to controls [120]. In contrast, patients with ataxia walk with an increased step width and larger ankle range of motion compared to controls, PD, and HSP [100]. Quantifying gait using wearable sensors is a valid measure for use with mild to moderate ataxia [26], with the mediolateral acceleration of the upper body during gait in particular being specific to disease and sensitive to symptom severity. Therefore, this may serve as a clinical biomarker for ataxia [122]. Gait outcomes extracted using more complex non-linear and data-driven approaches also offer potential, and are able to differentiate ataxias from other neurological patient groups [99,100,103]. Complex walking tasks such as incline walking [123], obstacle avoidance [124,125], and turning [102,122,126] may serve as 'stress tests' to exacerbate underlying gait impairments in ataxia and identify preclinical changes in this patient group [127].

3.3. Dementia

Dementia is a neurodegenerative syndrome that is characterised by multiple cognitive impairments affecting social and/or occupational functioning [128,129]. Globally, almost 50 million people are affected, the majority of whom are aged over 65. Risk increases exponentially with age, leading to high socioeconomic costs [130,131]. Dementia has many subtypes driven by different pathologies, the most common incorporating: Alzheimer's disease (AD); Lewy body dementias (LBD), which is comprised of dementia with Lewy bodies (DLB) and Parkinson's disease dementia (PDD); and vascular dementia (VaD). Mild cognitive impairment (MCI) may also be a risk factor for dementia, and can also be classified into subtypes [129,132]. The early and accurate identification of dementia and its subtype is of importance; however, it remains clinically challenging. Improved differentiation is critical, as misdiagnosis can lead to incorrect treatment and management of disease [133]. This is particularly pronounced between LBD and AD due to shared clinical features and cross-pathology [134–136]. DLB is pathologically classified by the presence of Lewy bodies containing abnormally folded alpha-synuclein within the brain. Clinically, it is differentiated from AD by prominent deficits in attention, visuospatial and executive function, cognitive fluctuations, visual hallucinations, RBD, and parkinsonism [133].

Gait, rather than being an autonomous task, is under cognitive control due to shared neural networks, and is evident in dementia cohorts [137]. Slow gait precedes and predicts cognitive decline and dementia, with gait impairments occurring up to nine years prior to diagnosis [138]. Even in the early stages of cognitive impairment, people with MCI walk slower, with shorter steps and increased variability compared to cognitively intact older adults [139,140]. People with dementia walk slower, with shorter strides and increased stride time variability compared to controls, and this increases with disease severity [140–144]. A recent review of gait across common dementia subtypes revealed slower gait and impaired timing (i.e., longer stance, stride, double support time) in people with AD, LBD, and VaD compared to controls [145–148], and demonstrated some evidence for a greater variability of gait in people with AD [149–153]. Falls risk is also increased in dementia and MCI, with DLB and PDD subtypes reporting the greatest risk [154]. An important link has been demonstrated in those with preclinical AD and falls, highlighting a possible underlying pathological basis, as amyloid burden predicted falls risk [155]. Discrete gait characteristics may serve as a useful tool for distinguishing between dementia subtypes [31], and can thus aid diagnosis. Differences between subtypes include slower gait in VaD compared to AD and slower pace, impaired timing, and an increased variability of gait in LBD compared to AD [145]. There is evidence to suggest that gait impairments differ across MCI subtypes [153], supporting a role for discrete gait outcomes as clinical biomarkers to aid diagnosis.

Only a small number of studies have looked at postural control in older adults with cognitive impairment, making it difficult to draw robust conclusions. A recent review reported impaired postural control in MCI [139] and AD [156]. However, group differences are not consistent [156]. More research may demonstrate postural control assessment, in addition to gait analysis, as a useful biomarker of cognitive impairment.

More recently, the monitoring of gait using body-worn sensors as in other neurological diseases has been explored in people with dementia. A recent study showed that clinic and home-based monitoring was feasible and acceptable in dementia populations, and trends suggest that gait impairments such as greater variability and a slower pace can differentiate dementia from controls when measured in free-living environments [157,158]. This shows potential use for monitoring gait prior to dementia onset and throughout the progression of the disease, providing valuable insight into the utility of gait as a clinical tool for the diagnosis and monitoring of dementia.

3.4. Summary

The current literature suggests that measuring gait and postural control has utility as a clinical tool, both for supporting diagnosis and monitoring disease progression. Impairments in gait and postural control may be the first manifestation of underlying neurological disease, such as in Parkinson's disease, ataxia, and dementia. There is evidence for the role of gait analysis in predicting and identifying the onset of cognitive decline in Parkinson's disease, and emerging evidence for the use of gait as a possible biomarker of dementia subtype. The early accurate diagnosis of these neurodegenerative conditions is a key target within clinical research, and the recent emergence of inexpensive wearable technology for analysing gait and posture has potential to be deployed as a widespread diagnostic tool. Quantifying gait and postural deficits can also be informative towards fall risk, which is a common problem in neurological conditions. Gait and postural measurements are increasingly used for disease progression monitoring, and may form an important part of a digital endpoint in clinical trials. Wearable technology and quantitative clinical measures may lead to improvements in the accurate identification of diagnosis, and may highlight individuals who would benefit from targeted intervention. Lastly, there is the opportunity to combine movement-based measures with biochemical and genetic analysis, such as in PD, where carriers of the autosomal dominant G2019S showed significant changes in gait variability compared to non-carriers [159].

4. Section III: Emerging Techniques for Disease Classification and Risk Prediction—So-Called 'Big Data' Approaches

It is evident that there is a plethora of measurement outcomes that are used to describe gait and postural control that are often used generally across a range of neurological conditions. Typically, a univariate approach is adopted, whereby measurement outcomes are considered independently, which may increase the risk of losing important information. Developing methods to reduce the number of (gait or postural) measurement outcomes included within statistical models is needed. Data-driven approaches that apply machine learning principles are beginning to explore the optimal combination of characteristics that successfully classify patients by condition (Figure 2) to improve diagnostic accuracy [160]. Recent work has used gait characteristics for fall classification in people with PD [161], and sensitivity analysis for feature selection when classifying PD [162]. A variety of data mining and machine learning approaches have been used to classify neurological conditions using gait and postural control data. For example, support vector machine techniques identified patients in the early stages of PD using their step length, which was measured during gait [163]. Multiple layer perception neural networks have distinguished Friedrich's ataxia from controls using stride time and gyroscope-derived outcomes [164]. Postural control measures have demonstrated utility for distinguishing AD from controls [165]. Adopting these analytical approaches also allow for gait and postural control outcomes to be considered in combination rather than independently. However, further research is required to select the appropriate gait and postural control characteristics for each disease type. This will aid clinical interpretation, reduce computational demand, and improve classification accuracy [12,166].

Realistically, in the future, wearable sensors will be the most practical tool to use to capture gait and postural control. However, gait and postural control data derived from wearable sensors is complex, multidimensional, and has high patient variability (no two patients are alike). Therefore, there is a need to find measures that offer increased sensitivity for distinguishing between neurological conditions at each disease severity level while controlling for between-person variability. Promising attempts to model and classify dementia and PD using measures of gait and postural control with a variety of classification tools (e.g., support vector machines, hidden Markov models, multilayer layer perception, neural networks, etc.) have been reported [163–165,167–171]. Even though the perfect classification accuracy is reported with various techniques, the optimal method or combination of approaches has not been identified, much less tested. In addition, robust modelling has not been possible, because studies are often limited to data collected in small, poorly described patient cohorts. Efficient systems for computational processing, the visualisation of multivariate gait and postural control profiles, and disease modelling in a clinician-friendly format are also essential for clinical adoption. There are currently no established tools for identifying and detecting disease or modelling disease progression in neurological diseases such as those described in this review. This is currently an area of significant interest.

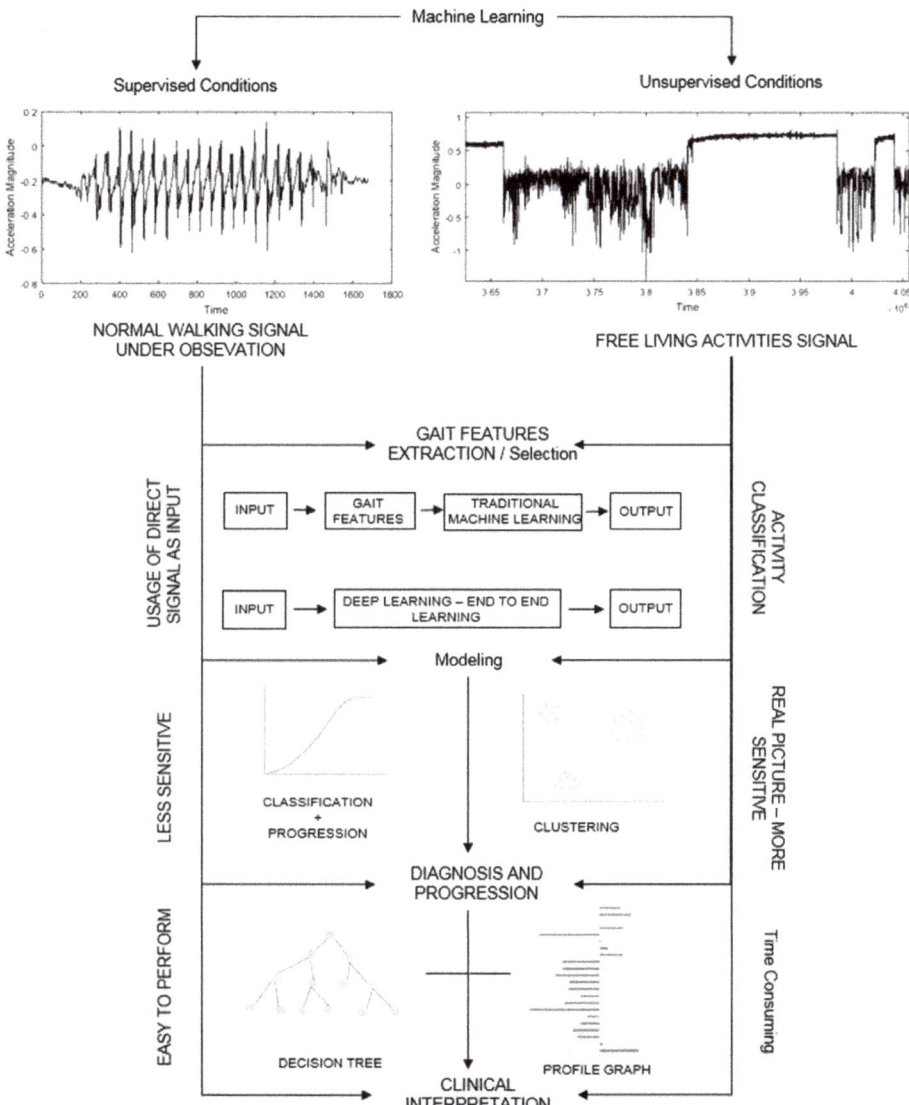

Figure 2. A machine learning end-to-end framework for the analysis of gait dynamics in the laboratory and community.

5. Section IV: Recommendations and Future Direction

A growing interest and body of literature is evident in the area of gait and postural control measurement. Complex techniques such as motion capture are unlikely to be deployed in clinical settings on a large scale in their present form due to their considerable cost, the dedicated personnel/expertise required, and potentially lengthy data collection and analysis period. However, techniques that reduce participant preparation time are currently being developed (i.e., markerless motion capture [172–174]) and aim to drive down financial cost, improve accessibility, reduce data collection time, and ultimately increase productivity. Although showing promise, similar to wearable sensors, research into the accuracy and validity of each device is paramount before integration in routine clinical practice. Furthermore, continued research should strive towards continued algorithm development to provide the most robust sensitive measures to clinicians so as to overcome the current pitfalls of the technology. The ultimate goal of community-based methods to quantify gait and postural control is to characterise clinical populations on a global scale and revolutionise current healthcare practises. Remote monitoring offers the opportunity to put the patient at the forefront of his or her own healthcare and management, and provide timely and effective intervention. First, to achieve such progress, it is imperative to ensure that the platform (device, outcomes, protocols, analytical pipelines, and processes) for collecting this information is robust, and personal data remains secure. This will allow the creation of normative databases, increasing prognostic capacity and providing a comprehensive understanding of the clinical landscape and therapeutic needs. Novel therapeutic interventions are required that are personalised, targeted to specific gait and postural impairments, and ultimately effective.

Future challenges include disentangling the process of ageing from the accelerated process of neurodegeneration whilst accounting for individual variation, comorbidities, lifestyle, overlapping sequelae, and atypical disorders, etc. To achieve this goal, the investigation of deep/machine learning techniques that have the potential to include other non-movement analysis-derived biomarkers appears to be a worthy pursuit. As such, more epidemiological studies are required to understand the interaction between lifestyle factors, individual capacity, and the environment [175] to improve prognostic and diagnostic accuracy. Collecting and aligning prodromal and disease cohort studies through dedicated consortia will enrich our current understanding of biomarkers and risk factors. Incorporating post mortem data retrospectively would be beneficial to verify the underlying pathology in complex conditions.

Recommendations

- Quantitative, objective assessments of gait and postural control should supplement traditional disease-specific scales in clinical trials to aid diagnostic accuracy and patient monitoring.
- Education around the advantages and disadvantages of quantitative analysis should be available to allow the clinician and clinical academic to make an informed decision about the best tool, protocol, and outcomes.
- Continued efforts are needed to validate the optimal protocol and outcome measures to best inform clinical management and research, and this requires a discrete condition-based approach.
- Further research using machine/deep learning should be explored to advance opportunities for optimised diagnosis and disease monitoring.
- Development of normative values across a range of standardised outcomes will help interpret gait and postural control outcome measures, and embed their clinical use and a personalised approach to management.
- Further research is needed in order to validate gait and postural control as approved disease biomarkers and progression markers.

Author Contributions: Conceptualisation, L.R.; Writing—Original draft preparation, C.B., L.A., R.M., R.Z.U.R., S.D.D., A.Y., C.M. and L.R.; Writing—Review and editing, L.R., L.A., C.B. and A.Y. Visualisation was contributed by C.B., L.A. and R.Z.U.R.

Funding: This research received no external funding.

Acknowledgments: The authors salaries are supported by the following: the National Institute for Health Research (NIHR) Newcastle Biomedical Research Centre (BRC) based at Newcastle upon Tyne Hospitals NHS Foundation Trust and Newcastle University; the NIHR Sheffield BRC; EU Horizon 2020 research and innovation programme under the Marie Skłodowska-Curie grant agreement No 721577; The Alzheimer's Society; The MRC and NIHR as part of Dementias Platform UK. The authors greatly appreciate and acknowledge the support provided.

Conflicts of Interest: The authors declare no conflict of interest.

References

1. Tinetti, M.E. Performance-oriented assessment of mobility problems in elderly patients. *J. Am. Geriatr. Soc.* **1986**, *34*, 119–126. [CrossRef]
2. Anne, S.-C.; Marjorie, H. *Motor Control: Theory and Practical Applications*; Lippincott, Williams & Wilkins: Philadelphia, PA, USA, 2000.
3. Berg, K.; Wood-Dauphine, S.; Williams, J.I.; Gayton, D. Measuring balance in the elderly: Preliminary development of an instrument. *Physiother. Can.* **1989**, *41*, 304–311. [CrossRef]
4. Berg, K.O.; Maki, B.E.; Williams, J.I.; Holliday, P.J.; Wood-Dauphinee, S.L. Clinical and laboratory measures of postural balance in an elderly population. *Arch. Phys. Med. Rehabil.* **1992**, *73*, 1073–1080. [PubMed]
5. Fritz, S.; Lusardi, M. Walking speed: The sixth vital sign. *J. Geriatr. Phys. Ther.* **2009**, *32*, 2–5. [CrossRef]
6. Cimolin, V.; Galli, M. Summary measures for clinical gait analysis: A literature review. *Gait Posture* **2014**, *39*, 1005–1010. [CrossRef] [PubMed]
7. Godinho, C.; Domingos, J.; Cunha, G.; Santos, A.T.; Fernandes, R.M.; Abreu, D.; Gonçalves, N.; Matthews, H.; Isaacs, T.; Duffen, J.; et al. A systematic review of the characteristics and validity of monitoring technologies to assess Parkinson's disease. *J. Neuroeng. Rehabil.* **2016**, *13*, 24. [CrossRef]
8. Ferrari, A.; Benedetti, M.G.; Pavan, E.; Frigo, C.; Bettinelli, D.; Rabuffetti, M.; Crenna, P.; Leardini, A. Quantitative comparison of five current protocols in gait analysis. *Gait Posture* **2008**, *28*, 207–216. [CrossRef]
9. Menz, H.B.; Latt, M.D.; Tiedemann, A.; Kwan, M.M.S.; Lord, S.R. Reliability of the GAITRite walkway system for the quantification of temporo-spatial parameters of gait in young and older people. *Gait Posture* **2004**, *20*, 20–25. [CrossRef]
10. Mcdonough, A.L.; Batavia, M.; Chen, F.C.; Kwon, S.; Ziai, J.; Al, A.M.; Batavia, M.; Fc, C. The Validity and Reliability of the GAITRite System's Measurements: A Preliminary Evaluation. *Arch. Phys. Med. Rehabil.* **2001**, *82*, 419–425. [CrossRef]
11. Van Uden, C.J.T.; Besser, M.P. Test-retest reliability of temporal and spatial gait characteristics measured with an instrumented walkway system (GAITRite). *BMC Musculoskelet. Disord.* **2004**, *5*, 13. [CrossRef]
12. Lord, S.; Galna, B.; Rochester, L. Moving forward on gait measurement: Toward a more refined approach. *Mov. Disord.* **2013**, *28*, 1534–1543. [CrossRef] [PubMed]
13. Galna, B.; Lord, S.; Rochester, L. Is gait variability reliable in older adults and Parkinson's disease? Towards an optimal testing protocol. *Gait Posture* **2013**, *37*, 580–585. [CrossRef] [PubMed]
14. Muro-De-La-Herran, A.; Garcia-Zapirain, B.; Mendez-Zorrilla, A. Gait analysis methods: An overview of wearable and non-wearable systems, highlighting clinical applications. *Sensors* **2014**, *14*, 3362–3394. [CrossRef] [PubMed]
15. Del Din, S.; Godfrey, A.; Mazza, C.; Lord, S.; Rochester, L. Free-Living Monitoring of Parkinson's Disease: Lessons from the Field. *Mov. Disord.* **2016**, *31*, 1293–1313. [CrossRef] [PubMed]
16. Weiss, A.; Sharifi, S.; Plotnik, M.; van Vugt, J.P.P.; Giladi, N.; Hausdorff, J.M. Toward Automated, At-Home Assessment of Mobility among Patients with Parkinson Disease, Using a Body-Worn Accelerometer. *Neurorehabil. Neural Repair* **2011**, *25*, 810–818. [CrossRef] [PubMed]
17. Weiss, A.; Brozgol, M.; Dorfman, M.; Herman, T.; Shema, S.; Giladi, N.; Hausdorff, J.M. Does the evaluation of gait quality during daily life provide insight into fall risk? A novel approach using 3-Day accelerometer recordings. *Neurorehabil. Neural Repair* **2013**, *27*, 742–752. [CrossRef]
18. Weiss, A.; Herman, T.; Giladi, N.; Hausdorff, J.M. Objective assessment of fall risk in Parkinson's disease using a body-fixed sensor worn for 3 days. *PLoS ONE* **2014**, *9*, e96675. [CrossRef]
19. Croce, U. Della; Cereatti, A.; Mancini, M. Gait Parameters Estimated Using Inertial Measurement Units. In *Handbook of Human Motion*; Springer: Cham, Switzerland, 2017.
20. Morris, R.; Hickey, A.; Del Din, S.; Godfrey, A.; Lord, S.; Rochester, L. A model of free-living gait: A factor analysis in Parkinson's disease. *Gait Posture* **2017**, *52*, 68–71. [CrossRef]
21. Lowe, S.A.; ÓLaighin, G. Monitoring human health behaviour in one's living environment: A technological review. *Med. Eng. Phys.* **2014**, *36*, 147–168. [CrossRef]
22. El-Gohary, M.; Pearson, S.; McNames, J.; Mancini, M.; Horak, F.; Mellone, S.; Chiari, L. Continuous monitoring of turning in patients with movement disability. *Sensors* **2014**, *14*, 356–369. [CrossRef]

23. Awais, M.; Palmerini, L.; Bourke, A.; Ihlen, E.; Helbostad, J.; Chiari, L. Performance Evaluation of State of the Art Systems for Physical Activity Classification of Older Subjects Using Inertial Sensors in a Real Life Scenario: A Benchmark Study. *Sensors* **2016**, *16*, 2105. [CrossRef] [PubMed]
24. Buckley, C.; Galna, B.; Rochester, L.; Mazzà, C. Upper body accelerations as a biomarker of gait impairment in the early stages of Parkinson's disease. *Gait Posture* **2018**. [CrossRef] [PubMed]
25. Del Din, S.; Godfrey, A.; Rochester, L. Validation of an Accelerometer to Quantify a Comprehensive Battery of Gait Characteristics in Healthy Older Adults and Parkinson's Disease: Toward Clinical and at Home Use. *IEEE J. Biomed. Health Inform.* **2016**, *20*, 838–847. [CrossRef] [PubMed]
26. Hickey, A.; Gunn, E.; Alcock, L.; Del Din, S.; Godfrey, A.; Rochester, L.; Galna, B. Validity of a wearable accelerometer to quantify gait in spinocerebellar ataxia type 6. *Physiol. Meas.* **2016**, *37*, N105–N117. [CrossRef]
27. Robles-García, V.; Corral-Bergantiños, Y.; Espinosa, N.; Jácome, M.A.; García-Sancho, C.; Cudeiro, J.; Arias, P. Spatiotemporal gait patterns during overt and covert evaluation in patients with Parkinson's disease and healthy subjects: Is there a Hawthorne effect? *J. Appl. Biomech.* **2015**, *31*, 189–194. [CrossRef]
28. Lord, S.; Galna, B.; Verghese, J.; Coleman, S.; Burn, D.; Rochester, L. Independent domains of gait in older adults and associated motor and nonmotor attributes: Validation of a factor analysis approach. *J. Gerontol. A. Biol. Sci. Med. Sci.* **2013**, *68*, 820–827. [CrossRef]
29. Beauchet, O.; Allali, G.; Sekhon, H.; Verghese, J.; Guilain, S.; Steinmetz, J.-P.; Kressig, R.W.; Barden, J.M.; Szturm, T.; Launay, C.P. Guidelines for assessment of gait and reference values for spatiotemporal gait parameters in older adults: The biomathics and canadian gait consortiums initiative. *Front. Hum. Neurosci.* **2017**, *11*, 353. [CrossRef]
30. Oh-Park, M.; Holtzer, R.; Xue, X.; Verghese, J. Conventional and robust quantitative gait norms in community-dwelling older adults. *J. Am. Geriatr. Soc.* **2010**, *58*, 1512–1518. [CrossRef]
31. Verghese, J.; Robbins, M.; Holtzer, R.; Zimmerman, M.; Wang, C.; Xue, X.; Lipton, R.B. Gait dysfunction in mild cognitive impairment syndromes. *J. Am. Geriatr. Soc.* **2008**, *56*, 1244–1251. [CrossRef]
32. Hollman, J.; McDade, E.; Petersen, R.C. Undefined Normative spatiotemporal gait parameters in older adults. *Gait Posture* **2011**, *34*, 111–118. [CrossRef]
33. Hausdorff, J.M. Gait variability: Methods, modeling and meaning Example of Increased Stride Time Variability in Elderly Fallers Quantification of Stride-to-Stride Fluctuations. *J. Neuroeng. Rehabil.* **2005**, *2*, 19. [CrossRef] [PubMed]
34. Hausdorff, J.M. Gait dynamics in Parkinson's disease: Common and distinct behavior among stride length, gait variability, and fractal-like scaling. *Chaos Interdiscip. J. Nonlinear Sci.* **2009**, *19*, 026113. [CrossRef] [PubMed]
35. Graham, J.E.; Ostir, G.V.; Fisher, S.R.; Ottenbacher, K.J. Assessing walking speed in clinical research: A systematic review. *J. Eval. Clin. Pract.* **2008**, *14*, 552–562. [CrossRef] [PubMed]
36. Van Kan, G.A.; Rolland, Y.; Andrieu, S.; Bauer, J.; Beauchet, O.; Bonnefoy, M.; Cesari, M.; Donini, L.M.; Gillette-Guyonnet, S.; Inzitari, M. Gait speed at usual pace as a predictor of adverse outcomes in community-dwelling older people an International Academy on Nutrition and Aging (IANA) Task Force. *J. Nutr. Health Aging* **2009**, *13*, 881–889. [CrossRef]
37. Lim, L.; Van Wegen, E.E.H.; De Goede, C.J.T.; Jones, D.; Rochester, L.; Hetherington, V.; Nieuwboer, A.; Willems, A.-M.; Kwakkel, G. Measuring gait and gait-related activities in Parkinson's patients own home environment: A reliability, responsiveness and feasibility study. *Parkinsonism Relat. Disord.* **2005**, *11*, 19–24. [CrossRef]
38. Steffen, T.; Seney, M. Test-retest reliability and minimal detectable change on balance and ambulation tests, the 36-item short-form health survey, and the unified Parkinson disease rating scale in people with parkinsonism. *Phys. Ther.* **2008**, *88*, 733–746. [CrossRef]
39. Ries, J.D.; Echternach, J.L.; Nof, L.; Gagnon Blodgett, M. Test-retest reliability and minimal detectable change scores for the timed "up & go" test, the six-minute walk test, and gait speed in people with Alzheimer disease. *Phys. Ther.* **2009**, *89*, 569–579. [CrossRef]
40. Tyson, S.; Connell, L. The psychometric properties and clinical utility of measures of walking and mobility in neurological conditions: A systematic review. *Clin. Rehabil.* **2009**, *23*, 1018–1033. [CrossRef]
41. Hollman, J.H.; Childs, K.B.; McNeil, M.L.; Mueller, A.C.; Quilter, C.M.; Youdas, J.W. Number of strides required for reliable measurements of pace, rhythm and variability parameters of gait during normal and dual task walking in older individuals. *Gait Posture* **2010**, *32*, 23–28. [CrossRef]

42. Riva, F.; Bisi, M.C.; Stagni, R. Gait variability and stability measures: Minimum number of strides and within-session reliability. *Comput. Biol. Med.* **2014**, *50*, 9–13. [CrossRef]
43. Steffen, T.M.; Hacker, T.A.; Mollinger, L. Age-and gender-related test performance in community-dwelling elderly people: Six-Minute Walk Test, Berg Balance Scale, Timed Up & Go Test, and gait speeds. *Phys. Ther.* **2002**, *82*, 128–137. [PubMed]
44. Snijders, A.H.; van de Warrenburg, B.P.; Giladi, N.; Bloem, B.R. Neurological gait disorders in elderly people: Clinical approach and classification. *Lancet Neurol.* **2007**, *6*, 63–74. [CrossRef]
45. Mancini, M.; Salarian, A.; Carlson-Kuhta, P.; Zampieri, C.; King, L.; Chiari, L.; Horak, F.B. ISway: A sensitive, valid and reliable measure of postural control. *J. Neuroeng. Rehabil.* **2012**, *9*, 59. [CrossRef] [PubMed]
46. Mancini, M.; Horak, F. Trunk accelerometry reveals postural instability in untreated Parkinson's disease. *Parkinsonism Relat. Disord.* **2011**, *17*, 557–562. [CrossRef] [PubMed]
47. Schoneburg, B.; Mancini, M. Framework for understanding balance dysfunction in Parkinson's disease. *Mov. Disord.* **2013**, *28*, 1474–1482. [CrossRef] [PubMed]
48. Baston, C.; Mancini, M.; Schoneburg, B.; Horak, F.; Rocchi, L. Postural strategies assessed with inertial sensors in healthy and parkinsonian subjects. *Gait Posture* **2014**, *40*, 70–75. [CrossRef] [PubMed]
49. Kelly, V.E.; Johnson, C.O.; McGough, E.L.; Shumway-Cook, A.; Horak, F.B.; Chung, K.A.; Espay, A.J.; Revilla, F.J.; Devoto, J.; Wood-Siverio, C. Association of cognitive domains with postural instability/gait disturbance in Parkinson's disease. *Parkinsonism Relat. Disord.* **2015**, *21*, 692–697. [CrossRef] [PubMed]
50. Rocchi, L.; Chiari, L.; Horak, F.B. Effects of deep brain stimulation and levodopa on postural sway in Parkinson's disease. *J. Neurol. Neurosurg. Psychiatry* **2002**, *73*, 267–274. [CrossRef]
51. Palmerini, L.; Rocchi, L.; Mellone, S.; Valzania, F.; Chiari, L. Feature selection for accelerometer-based posture analysis in Parkinsons disease. *IEEE Trans. Inf. Technol. Biomed.* **2011**, *15*, 481–490. [CrossRef]
52. Fukunaga, J.Y.; Quitschal, R.M.; Doná, F.; Ferraz, H.B.; Ganança, M.M.; Caovilla, H.H. Postural control in Parkinson's disease. *Braz. J. Otorhinolaryngol.* **2014**, *80*, 508–514. [CrossRef]
53. Pantall, A.; Del, S.; Rochester, L. Longitudinal changes over thirty-six months in postural control dynamics and cognitive function in people with Parkinson's disease. *Gait Posture* **2018**, *62*, 468–474. [CrossRef] [PubMed]
54. Ruhe, A.; Fejer, R.; Walker, B. The test-retest reliability of centre of pressure measures in bipedal static task conditions–a systematic review of the literature. *Gait Posture* **2010**, *32*, 436–445. [CrossRef]
55. Mancini, M.; Horak, F.B. The relevance of clinical balance assessment tools to differentiate balance deficits. *Eur. J. Phys. Rehabil. Med.* **2010**, *46*, 239. [PubMed]
56. Del Din, S.; Godfrey, A.; Coleman, S.; Galna, B.; Lord, S.; Rochester, L. Time-dependent changes in postural control in early Parkinson's disease: What are we missing? *Med. Biol. Eng. Comput.* **2016**, *54*, 401–410. [CrossRef] [PubMed]
57. Paillard, T.; Noé, F. Techniques and Methods for Testing the Postural Function in Healthy and Pathological Subjects. *BioMed Res. Int.* **2015**, 981390. [CrossRef]
58. Dorsey, E.R.; Bloem, B.R. The Parkinson pandemic—A call to action. *JAMA Neurol.* **2018**, *75*, 9–10. [CrossRef]
59. Feigin, V.L.; Abajobir, A.A.; Abate, K.H.; Abd-Allah, F.; Abdulle, A.M.; Abera, S.F.; Abyu, G.Y.; Ahmed, M.B.; Aichour, A.N.; Aichour, I. Global, regional, and national burden of neurological disorders during 1990-2015: A systematic analysis for the Global Burden of Disease Study 2015. *Lancet Neurol.* **2017**, *16*, 877–897. [CrossRef]
60. Emamzadeh, F.N.; Surguchov, A. Parkinson's Disease: Biomarkers, Treatment, and Risk Factors. *Front. Neurosci.* **2018**, *12*, 612. [CrossRef]
61. Marinus, J.; Zhu, K.; Marras, C.; Aarsland, D.; van Hilten, J.J. Risk factors for non-motor symptoms in Parkinson's disease. *Lancet Neurol.* **2018**, *17*, 559–568. [CrossRef]
62. Goetz, C.G.; Tilley, B.C.; Shaftman, S.R.; Stebbins, G.T.; Fahn, S.; Martinez-Martin, P.; Poewe, W.; Sampaio, C.; Stern, M.B.; Dodel, R. Movement Disorder Society-sponsored revision of the Unified Parkinson's Disease Rating Scale (MDS-UPDRS): Scale presentation and clinimetric testing results. *Mov. Disord.* **2008**, *23*, 2129–2170. [CrossRef]
63. Hoehn, M.M.; Yahr, M.D. Parkinsonism: Onset, progression, and mortality. *Neurology* **1967**, *17*, 427. [CrossRef] [PubMed]
64. Rovini, E.; Maremmani, C.; Cavallo, F. How wearable sensors can support parkinson's disease diagnosis and treatment: A systematic review. *Front. Neurosci.* **2017**, *11*, 555. [CrossRef] [PubMed]

65. Galna, B.; Lord, S.; Burn, D.J.; Rochester, L. Progression of Gait Dysfunction in Incident Parkinson's Disease: Impact of Medication and Phenotype. *Mov. Disord.* **2015**, *30*, 359–367. [CrossRef] [PubMed]
66. Jankovic, J. Parkinson's disease: Clinical features and diagnosis. *J. Neurol. Neurosurg. Psychiatry* **2008**, *79*, 368–376. [CrossRef]
67. Schaafsma, J.D.; Giladi, N.; Balash, Y.; Bartels, A.L.; Gurevich, T.; Hausdorff, J.M. Gait dynamics in Parkinson's disease: Relationship to Parkinsonian features, falls and response to levodopa. *J. Neurol. Sci.* **2003**, *212*, 47–53. [CrossRef]
68. Hoskovcová, M.; Dusek, P.; Sieger, T.; Brozová, H.; Zárubová, K.; Bezdicek, O.; Sprdlik, O.; Jech, R.; Stochl, J.; Roth, J.; et al. Predicting falls in Parkinson disease: What is the value of instrumented testing in off medication state? *PLoS ONE* **2015**, *10*, e0139849. [CrossRef]
69. Morris, R.; Lord, S.; Lawson, R.A.; Coleman, S.; Galna, B.; Duncan, G.W.; Khoo, T.K.; Yarnall, A.J.; Burn, D.J.; Rochester, L. Gait Rather Than Cognition Predicts Decline in Specific Cognitive Domains in Early Parkinson's Disease. *J. Gerontol. Ser. A* **2017**, *72*, 1656–1662. [CrossRef]
70. Coelho, M.; Ferreira, J.J. Late-stage Parkinson disease. *Nat. Rev. Neurol.* **2012**, *8*, 435. [CrossRef]
71. Rochester, L.; Galna, B.; Lord, S.; Yarnall, A.J.; Morris, R.; Duncan, G.; Khoo, T.K.; Mollenhauer, B.; Burn, D.J. Decrease in Aβ42 predicts dopa-resistant gait progression in early Parkinson disease. *Neurology* **2017**, *88*, 1501–1511. [CrossRef]
72. McDade, E.M.; Boot, B.P.; Christianson, T.J.H.; Pankratz, V.S.; Boeve, B.F.; Ferman, T.J.; Bieniek, K.; Hollman, J.H.; Roberts, R.O.; Mielke, M.M.; et al. Subtle gait changes in patients with REM sleep behavior disorder. *Mov. Disord.* **2013**, *28*, 1847–1853. [CrossRef]
73. Lowry, K. a; Smiley-Oyen, A.L.; Carrel, A.J.; Kerr, J.P. Walking stability using harmonic ratios in Parkinson's disease. *Mov. Disord.* **2009**, *24*, 261–267. [CrossRef] [PubMed]
74. Latt, M.; Menz, H.; Fung, V.; Lord, S. Acceleration patterns of the head and pelvis during gait in older people with Parkinson's disease: A comparison of fallers and nonfallers. *J. Gerontol.* **2009**, *64*, 700–706. [CrossRef]
75. Latt, M.; Menz, H.; Fung, V.; Lord, S. Walking speed, cadence and step length are selected to optimize the stability of head and pelvis accelerations. *Exp. Brain Res.* **2008**, *184*, 201–209. [CrossRef]
76. Sejdic, E.; Lowry, K.; Roche, J.; Redfern, M.; Brach, J. A comprehensive assessment of gait accelerometry signals in time, frequency and time-frequency domains. *IEEE Trans. Neural Syst. Rehabil. Eng.* **2013**, *22*, 603–612. [CrossRef] [PubMed]
77. Mirelman, A.; Bernad-Elazari, H.; Thaler, A.; Giladi-Yacobi, E.; Gurevich, T.; Gana-Weisz, M.; Saunders-Pullman, R.; Raymond, D.; Doan, N.; Bressman, S.B. Arm swing as a potential new prodromal marker of Parkinson's disease. *Mov. Disord.* **2016**, *31*, 1527–1534. [CrossRef]
78. Rizzo, G.; Copetti, M.; Arcuti, S.; Martino, D.; Fontana, A.; Logroscino, G. Accuracy of clinical diagnosis of Parkinson disease A systematic review and meta-analysis. *Neurology* **2016**, *86*, 566–576. [CrossRef] [PubMed]
79. Smulders, K.; Dale, M.L.; Carlson-Kuhta, P.; Nutt, J.G.; Horak, F.B. Pharmacological treatment in Parkinson's disease: Effects on gait. *Parkinsonism Relat. Disord.* **2016**, *31*, 3–13. [CrossRef]
80. Rochester, L.; Yarnall, A.J.; Baker, M.R.; David, R.V.; Lord, S.; Galna, B.; Burn, D.J. Cholinergic dysfunction contributes to gait disturbance in early Parkinson's disease. *Brain* **2012**, *135*, 2779–2788. [CrossRef]
81. Muller, M.; Bohnen, N.; Bhaumik, A.; Albin, R.; Frey, K.; Gilman, S. Striatal dopaminergic denervation and cardiac post-ganglionic sympathetic denervation correlate independently with gait velocity in Parkinson disease. In *Neurology*; Lippincott Williams & Wilkins: Philadelphia, PA, USA, 2011; Volume 76, p. A265.
82. Bloem, B.; Hausdorff, J. Falls and freezing of gait in Parkinson's disease: A review of two interconnected, episodic phenomena. *Mov. Disord.* **2004**, *19*, 871–884. [CrossRef]
83. Shah, J.; Pillai, L.; Williams, D.K.; Doerhoff, S.M.; Larson-Prior, L.; Garcia-Rill, E.; Virmani, T. Increased foot strike variability in Parkinson's disease patients with freezing of gait. *Parkinsonism Relat. Disord.* **2018**, *53*, 58–63. [CrossRef]
84. Weiss, A.; Herman, T.; Giladi, N.; Hausdorff, J.M. New evidence for gait abnormalities among Parkinson's disease patients who suffer from freezing of gait: Insights using a body-fixed sensor worn for 3 days. *J. Neural Transm.* **2015**, *122*, 403–410. [CrossRef] [PubMed]
85. Hausdorff, J.M.; Schaafsma, J.D.; Balash, Y.; Bartels, A.L.; Gurevich, T.; Giladi, N. Impaired regulation of stride variability in Parkinson's disease subjects with freezing of gait. *Exp. Brain Res.* **2003**, *149*, 187–194. [CrossRef]

86. Moore, S.T.; Yungher, D.A.; Morris, T.R.; Dilda, V.; MacDougall, H.G.; Shine, J.M.; Naismith, S.L.; Lewis, S.J.G. Autonomous identification of freezing of gait in Parkinson's disease from lower-body segmental accelerometry. *J. Neuroeng. Rehabil.* **2013**, *10*, 19. [CrossRef] [PubMed]
87. Lipsmeier, F.; Taylor, K.I.; Kilchenmann, T.; Wolf, D.; Scotland, A.; Schjodt-Eriksen, J.; Cheng, W.-Y.; Fernandez-Garcia, I.; Siebourg-Polster, J.; Jin, L.; et al. Evaluation of smartphone-based testing to generate exploratory outcome measures in a phase 1 Parkinson's disease clinical trial. *Mov. Disord.* **2018**, *33*, 1287–1297. [CrossRef]
88. Rocchi, L.; Palmerini, L.; Weiss, A.; Herman, T.; Hausdorff, J. Balance Testing With Inertial Sensors in Patients With Parkinson's Disease: Assessment of Motor Subtypes. *IEEE Trans. Neural Syst. Rehabil. Eng.* **2014**, *22*, 1064–1071. [CrossRef]
89. Oyama-Higa, M.; Niwa, T.; Wang, W.; Kawanabe, Y. Identifying Characteristic Physiological Patterns of Parkinson's Disease Sufferers using Sample Entropy of Pulse Waves. In Proceedings of the 11th International Joint Conference on Biomedical Engineering Systems and Technologies, Funchal, Portugal; 2018; pp. 189–196. [CrossRef]
90. Ruano, L.; Melo, C.; Silva, M.C.; Coutinho, P. The global epidemiology of hereditary ataxia and spastic paraplegia: A systematic review of prevalence studies. *Neuroepidemiology* **2014**, *42*, 174–183. [CrossRef] [PubMed]
91. Matsumura, R.; Futamura, N.; Fujimoto, Y.; Yanagimoto, S.; Horikawa, H.; Suzumura, A.; Takayanagi, T. Spinocerebellar ataxia type 6. Molecular and clinical features of 35 Japanese patients including one homozygous for the CAG repeat expansion. *Neurology* **1997**, *49*, 1238–1243. [CrossRef]
92. Furtado, S.; Das, S.; Suchowersky, O. A review of the inherited ataxias: Recent advances in genetic, clinical and neuropathologic aspects. *Park. Relat. Disord.* **1998**, *4*, 161–169. [CrossRef]
93. Takahashi, H.; Ishikawa, K.; Tsutsumi, T.; Fujigasaki, H.; Kawata, A.; Okiyama, R.; Fujita, T.; Yoshizawa, K.; Yamaguchi, S.; Tomiyasu, H. A clinical and genetic study in a large cohort of patients with spinocerebellar ataxia type 6. *J. Hum. Genet.* **2004**, *49*, 256. [CrossRef]
94. Globas, C.; du Montcel, S.T.; Baliko, L.; Boesch, S.; Depondt, C.; DiDonato, S.; Durr, A.; Filla, A.; Klockgether, T.; Mariotti, C. Early symptoms in spinocerebellar ataxia type 1, 2, 3, and 6. *Mov. Disord.* **2008**, *23*, 2232–2238. [CrossRef] [PubMed]
95. Rochester, L.; Galna, B.; Lord, S.; Mhiripiri, D.; Eglon, G.; Chinnery, P.F. Gait impairment precedes clinical symptoms in spinocerebellar ataxia type 6. *Mov. Disord.* **2014**, *29*, 252–255. [CrossRef] [PubMed]
96. Sakakibara, R.; Terayama, K.; Ogawa, A.; Haruta, H.; Akiba, T.; Tateno, F.; Kishi, M.; Tsuyusaki, Y.; Aiba, Y.; Ogata, T. Wearable gait sensors to measure degenerative cerebellar ataxia. *J. Neurol. Sci.* **2017**, *381*, 56–57. [CrossRef]
97. König, N.; Taylor, W.R.; Baumann, C.R.; Wenderoth, N.; Singh, N.B. Revealing the quality of movement: A meta-analysis review to quantify the thresholds to pathological variability during standing and walking. *Neurosci. Biobehav. Rev.* **2016**, *68*, 111–119. [CrossRef] [PubMed]
98. Pradhan, C.; Wuehr, M.; Akrami, F.; Neuhaeusser, M.; Huth, S.; Brandt, T.; Jahn, K.; Schniepp, R. Automated classification of neurological disorders of gait using spatio-temporal gait parameters. *J. Electromyogr. Kinesiol.* **2015**, *25*, 413–422. [CrossRef] [PubMed]
99. Chini, G.; Ranavolo, A.; Draicchio, F.; Casali, C.; Conte, C.; Martino, G.; Leonardi, L.; Padua, L.; Coppola, G.; Pierelli, F.; et al. Local Stability of the Trunk in Patients with Degenerative Cerebellar Ataxia During Walking. *Cerebellum* **2017**, *16*, 26–33. [CrossRef] [PubMed]
100. Serrao, M.; Chini, G.; Bergantino, M.; Sarnari, D.; Casali, C.; Conte, C.; Ranavolo, A.; Marcotulli, C.; Rinaldi, M.; Coppola, G.; et al. Identification of specific gait patterns in patients with cerebellar ataxia, spastic paraplegia, and Parkinson's disease: A non-hierarchical cluster analysis. *Hum. Mov. Sci.* **2018**, *57*, 267–279. [CrossRef]
101. Buckley, E.; Mazzà, C.; McNeill, A. A systematic review of the gait characteristics associated with Cerebellar Ataxia. *Gait Posture* **2018**, *60*, 154–163. [CrossRef]
102. Serrao, M.; Mari, S.; Conte, C.; Ranavolo, A.; Casali, C.; Draicchio, F.; Di Fabio, R.; Bartolo, M.; Monamì, S.; Padua, L.; et al. Strategies adopted by cerebellar ataxia patients to perform u-turns. *Cerebellum* **2013**, *12*, 460–468. [CrossRef]

103. Serrao, M.; Chini, G.; Iosa, M.; Casali, C.; Morone, G.; Conte, C.; Bini, F.; Marinozzi, F.; Coppola, G.; Pierelli, F.; et al. Corrigendum to "Harmony as a convergence attractor that minimizes the energy expenditure and variability in physiological gait and the loss of harmony in cerebellar ataxia."[Clin. Biomech. 48 (2017) 15-23]. *Clin. Biomech.* **2017**, *50*, 160. [CrossRef]
104. Martino, G.; Ivanenko, Y.P.; Serrao, M.; Ranavolo, A.; d'Avella, A.; Draicchio, F.; Conte, C.; Casali, C.; Lacquaniti, F. Locomotor patterns in cerebellar ataxia. *J. Neurophysiol.* **2014**, *112*, 2810–2821. [CrossRef]
105. Sharma, J.; Maclennan, W. Causes of Ataxia in patients attending a falls laboratory. *Age Ageing* **1988**, *17*, 94–102. [CrossRef]
106. Schniepp, R.; Wuehr, M.; Neuhaeusser, M.; Kamenova, M.; Dimitriadis, K.; Klopstock, T.; Strupp, M.; Brandt, T.; Jahn, K. Locomotion speed determines gait variability in cerebellar ataxia and vestibular failure. *Mov. Disord.* **2012**, *27*, 125–131. [CrossRef] [PubMed]
107. Milne, S.C.; Murphy, A.; Georgiou-Karistianis, N.; Yiu, E.M.; Delatycki, M.B.; Corben, L.A. Psychometric properties of outcome measures evaluating decline in gait in cerebellar ataxia: A systematic review. *Gait Posture* **2018**, *61*, 149–162. [CrossRef] [PubMed]
108. Marquer, A.; Barbieri, G.; Pérennou, D. The assessment and treatment of postural disorders in cerebellar ataxia: A systematic review. *Ann. Phys. Rehabil. Med.* **2014**, *57*, 67–78. [CrossRef] [PubMed]
109. Stolze, H.; Klebe, S.; Baecker, C.; Zechlin, C.; Friege, L.; Pohle, S.; Deuschl, G. Prevalence of Gait disorders in hospitalized neurological patients. *Mov. Disord.* **2005**, *20*, 89–94. [CrossRef]
110. Jayadev, S.; Bird, T.D. Hereditary ataxias: Overview. *Genet. Med.* **2013**, *15*, 673–683. [CrossRef]
111. Sandford, E.; Burmeister, M. Genes and genetic testing in hereditary ataxias. *Genes* **2014**, *5*, 586–603. [CrossRef]
112. Schmitz-Hübsch, T.; Du Montcel, S.T.; Baliko, L.; Berciano, J.; Boesch, S.; Depondt, C.; Giunti, P.; Globas, C.; Infante, J.; Kang, J.-S. Scale for the assessment and rating of ataxia: Development of a new clinical scale. *Neurology* **2006**, *66*, 1717–1720. [CrossRef]
113. Ilg, W.; Golla, H.; Thier, P.; Giese, M.A. Specific influences of cerebellar dysfunctions on gait. *Brain* **2007**, *130*, 786–798. [CrossRef] [PubMed]
114. Comber, L.; Sosnoff, J.J.; Galvin, R.; Coote, S. Postural control deficits in people with Multiple Sclerosis: A systematic review and meta-analysis. *Gait Posture* **2018**, *61*, 445–452. [CrossRef] [PubMed]
115. Bakker, M.; Allum, J.H.J.; Visser, J.E.; Grüneberg, C.; van de Warrenburg, B.P.; Kremer, B.H.P.; Bloem, B.R. Postural responses to multidirectional stance perturbations in cerebellar ataxia. *Exp. Neurol.* **2006**, *202*, 21–35. [CrossRef] [PubMed]
116. Bunn, L.M.; Marsden, J.F.; Giunti, P.; Day, B.L. Stance instability in spinocerebellar ataxia type 6. *Mov. Disord.* **2013**, *28*, 510–516. [CrossRef] [PubMed]
117. Fonteyn, E.M.R.; Schmitz-Hübsch, T.; Verstappen, C.C.; Baliko, L.; Bloem, B.R.; Boesch, S.; Bunn, L.; Charles, P.; Dürr, A.; Filla, A.; et al. Falls in spinocerebellar ataxias: Results of the EuroSCA fall study. *Cerebellum* **2010**, *9*, 232–239. [CrossRef] [PubMed]
118. Paquette, C.; Franzén, E.; Horak, F.B. More falls in cerebellar ataxia when standing on a slow up- moving tilt of the support surface HHS Public Access. *Cerebellum* **2016**, *15*, 336–342. [CrossRef]
119. Van de Warrenburg, B.P.C.; Bakker, M.; Kremer, B.P.H.; Bloem, B.R.; Allum, J.H.J. Trunk sway in patients with spinocerebellar ataxia. *Mov. Disord.* **2005**, *20*, 1006–1013. [CrossRef] [PubMed]
120. Ramakers, R.; Koene, S.; Groothuis, J.T.; de Laat, P.; Janssen, M.C.H.; Smeitink, J. Quantification of gait in mitochondrial m. 3243A > G patients: A validation study. *Orphanet J. Rare Dis.* **2017**, *12*, 91. [CrossRef] [PubMed]
121. Serrao, M.; Chini, G.; Bergantino, M.; Sarnari, D.; Casali, C.; Conte, C.; Ranavolo, A.; Marcotulli, C.; Rinaldi, M.; Coppola, G. Dataset on gait patterns in degenerative neurological diseases. *Data Br.* **2018**, *16*, 806–816. [CrossRef]
122. Shirai, S.; Yabe, I.; Matsushima, M.; Ito, Y.M.; Yoneyama, M.; Sasaki, H. Quantitative evaluation of gait ataxia by accelerometers. *J. Neurol. Sci.* **2015**, *358*, 253–258. [CrossRef] [PubMed]
123. Earhart, G.M.; Bastian, A.J. Selection and coordination of human locomotor forms following cerebellar damage. *J. Neurophysiol.* **2001**, *85*, 759–769. [CrossRef]
124. Fonteyn, E.M.R.; Heeren, A.; Engels, J.J.C.; Den Boer, J.J.; van de Warrenburg, B.P.C.; Weerdesteyn, V. Gait adaptability training improves obstacle avoidance and dynamic stability in patients with cerebellar degeneration. *Gait Posture* **2014**, *40*, 247–251. [CrossRef]

125. Morton, S.M.; Dordevic, G.S.; Bastian, A.J. Cerebellar damage produces context-dependent deficits in control of leg dynamics during obstacle avoidance. *Exp. Brain Res.* **2004**, *156*, 149–163. [CrossRef] [PubMed]
126. Mari, S.; Serrao, M.; Casali, C.; Conte, C.; Ranavolo, A.; Padua, L.; Draicchio, F.; Iavicoli, S.; Monamì, S.; Sandrini, G.; et al. Turning strategies in patients with cerebellar ataxia. *Exp. Brain Res.* **2012**, *222*, 65–75. [CrossRef] [PubMed]
127. Ilg, W.; Fleszar, Z.; Schatton, C.; Hengel, H.; Harmuth, F.; Bauer, P.; Timmann, D.; Giese, M.; Schöls, L.; Synofzik, M. I ndividual changes in preclinical spinocerebellar ataxia identified via increased motor complexity. *Mov. Disord.* **2016**, *31*, 1891–1900. [CrossRef] [PubMed]
128. Alzheimer's Association. 2017 Alzheimer's disease facts and figures. *Alzheimers Dement.* **2017**, *13*, 325–373. [CrossRef]
129. American Psychiatric Association. *Diagnostic and Statistical Manual of Mental Disorders (DSM-5®)*; American Psychiatric Pub: New York, NY, USA, 2013; ISBN 0890425574.
130. Werner, P.; Savva, G.M.; Maidment, I.; Thyrian, J.R.; Fox, C. Dementia: Introduction, Epidemiology and Economic Impact. In *Mental Health and Older People*; Springer: Cham, Switzerland, 2016; pp. 197–209.
131. Prince, M.; Wimo, A.; Guerchet, M.; Ali, G.; Wu, Y.; Prina, M. *World Alzheimer Report 2015 The Global Impact of Dementia*; King's College: London, UK, 2015.
132. Gauthier, S.; Reisberg, B.; Zaudig, M.; Petersen, R.C.; Ritchie, K.; Broich, K.; Belleville, S.; Brodaty, H.; Bennett, D.; Chertkow, H. Mild cognitive impairment. *Lancet* **2006**, *367*, 1262–1270. [CrossRef]
133. Kane, J.P.M.; Surendranathan, A.; Bentley, A.; Barker, S.A.H.; Taylor, J.-P.; Thomas, A.J.; Allan, L.M.; McNally, R.J.; James, P.W.; McKeith, I.G.; et al. Clinical prevalence of Lewy body dementia. *Alzheimers. Res.* **2018**, *10*, 19. [CrossRef] [PubMed]
134. Toledo, J.B.; Cairns, N.J.; Da, X.; Chen, K.; Carter, D.; Fleisher, A.; Householder, E.; Ayutyanont, N.; Roontiva, A.; Bauer, R.J.; et al. Clinical and multimodal biomarker correlates of ADNI neuropathological findings. *Acta Neuropathol. Commun.* **2013**, *1*, 65. [CrossRef] [PubMed]
135. Tiraboschi, P.; Salmon, D.P.; Hansen, L.A.; Hofstetter, R.C.; Thal, L.J.; Corey-Bloom, J. What best differentiates Lewy body from Alzheimer's disease in early-stage dementia? *Brain* **2006**, *129*, 729–735. [CrossRef] [PubMed]
136. McKeith, I. Dementia with Lewy bodies. In *Handbook of Clinical Neurology*; Elsevier: Philadelphia, PA, USA, 2007; Volume 84, pp. 531–548.
137. Morris, R.; Lord, S.; Bunce, J.; Burn, D.; Rochester, L. Gait and cognition: Mapping the global and discrete relationships in ageing and neurodegenerative disease. *Neurosci. Biobehav. Rev.* **2016**, *64*, 326–345. [CrossRef]
138. Beauchet, O.; Annweiler, C.; Callisaya, M.L.; De Cock, A.-M.; Helbostad, J.L.; Kressig, R.W.; Srikanth, V.; Steinmetz, J.-P.; Blumen, H.M.; Verghese, J. Poor gait performance and prediction of dementia: Results from a meta-analysis. *J. Am. Med. Dir. Assoc.* **2016**, *17*, 482–490. [CrossRef]
139. Bahureksa, L.; Najafi, B.; Saleh, A.; Sabbagh, M.; Coon, D.; Mohler, M.J.; Schwenk, M. The impact of mild cognitive impairment on gait and balance: A systematic review and meta-analysis of studies using instrumented assessment. *Gerontology* **2017**, *63*, 67–83. [CrossRef] [PubMed]
140. Valkanova, V.; Ebmeier, K.P. What can gait tell us about dementia? Review of epidemiological and neuropsychological evidence. *Gait Posture* **2017**, *53*, 215–223. [CrossRef] [PubMed]
141. van Iersel, M.B.; Hoefsloot, W.; Munneke, M.; Bloem, B.R.; Rikkert, M.G.M.O. Systematic review of quantitative clinical gait analysis in patients with dementia. *Z. Gerontol. Geriatr.* **2004**, *37*, 27–32. [CrossRef] [PubMed]
142. Gillain, S.; Warzee, E.; Lekeu, F.; Wojtasik, V.; Maquet, D.; Croisier, J.L.; Salmon, E.; Petermans, J. The value of instrumental gait analysis in elderly healthy, MCI or Alzheimer's disease subjects and a comparison with other clinical tests used in single and dual-task conditions. *Ann. Phys. Rehabil. Med.* **2009**, *52*, 453–474. [CrossRef] [PubMed]
143. Coelho, F.G.; Stella, F.; de Andrade, L.P.; Barbieri, F.A.; Santos-Galduroz, R.F.; Gobbi, S.; Costa, J.L.; Gobbi, L.T. Gait and risk of falls associated with frontal cognitive functions at different stages of Alzheimer's disease. *Aging Neuropsychol. Cognit.* **2012**, *19*, 644–656. [CrossRef] [PubMed]
144. Muir, S.W.; Speechley, M.; Wells, J.; Borrie, M.; Gopaul, K.; Montero-Odasso, M. Gait assessment in mild cognitive impairment and Alzheimer's disease: The effect of dual-task challenges across the cognitive spectrum. *Gait Posture* **2012**, *35*, 96–100. [CrossRef] [PubMed]

145. Mc Ardle, R.; Morris, R.; Wilson, J.; Galna, B.; Thomas, A.J.; Rochester, L. What Can Quantitative Gait Analysis Tell Us about Dementia and Its Subtypes? A Structured Review. *J. Alzheimers Dis.* **2017**, *60*, 1295–1312. [CrossRef] [PubMed]
146. Fritz, N.E.; Kegelmeyer, D.A.; Kloos, A.D.; Linder, S.; Park, A.; Kataki, M.; Adeli, A.; Agrawal, P.; Scharre, D.W.; Kostyk, S.K. Motor Performance Differentiates Individuals with Lewy Body Dementia, Parkinson's and Alzheimer's Disease. *Gait Posture* **2016**, *50*, 1–7. [CrossRef] [PubMed]
147. Merory, J.R.; Wittwer, J.E.; Rowe, C.C.; Webster, K.E. Quantitative gait analysis in patients with dementia with Lewy bodies and Alzheimer's disease. *Gait Posture* **2007**, *26*, 414–419. [CrossRef] [PubMed]
148. Tanaka, A.; Okuzumi, H.; Kobayashi, I.; Murai, N.; Meguro, K.; Nakamura, T. Gait Disturbance of Patients with Vascular and Alzheimer-Type Dementias. *Percept. Mot. Ski.* **1995**, *80*, 735–738. [CrossRef] [PubMed]
149. Nakamura, T.; Meguro, K.; Sasaki, H. Relationship between falls and stride length variability in senile dementia of the Alzheimer type. *Gerontology* **1996**, *42*, 108–113. [CrossRef] [PubMed]
150. Webster, K.E.; Merory, J.R.; Wittwer, J.E. Gait Variability in Community Dwelling Adults With Alzheimer Disease. *Alzheimer Dis. Assoc. Disord.* **2006**, *20*, 37–40. [CrossRef] [PubMed]
151. Maquet, D.; Lekeu, F.; Warzee, E.; Gillain, S.; Wojtasik, V.; Salmon, E.; Petermans, J.; Croisier, J.L. Gait analysis in elderly adult patients with mild cognitive impairment and patients with mild Alzheimer's disease: Simple versus dual task: A preliminary report. *Clin. Physiol. Funct. Imaging* **2010**, *30*, 51–56. [CrossRef] [PubMed]
152. Western Geriatric Research Institute. *Alzheimer Disease and Associated Disorders*; Lawrence, K., Ed.; Western Geriatric Research Institute: Philadelphia, PA, USA, 1987.
153. Allali, G.; Annweiler, C.; Blumen, H.M.; Callisaya, M.L.; De Cock, A.-M.M.; Kressig, R.W.; Srikanth, V.; Steinmetz, J.-P.P.; Verghese, J.; Beauchet, O. Gait phenotype from mild cognitive impairment to moderate dementia: Results from the GOOD initiative. *Eur. J. Neurol.* **2016**, *23*, 527–541. [CrossRef] [PubMed]
154. Rochester, L.; Lord, S.; Yarnall, A.J.; Burn, D.J. Falls in Patients with Dementia. In *Movement Disorders in Dementias*; Springer: London, UK, 2014; pp. 45–60.
155. Stark, S.L.; Roe, C.M.; Grant, E.A.; Hollingsworth, H.; Benzinger, T.L.; Fagan, A.M.; Buckles, V.D.; Morris, J.C. Preclinical Alzheimer disease and risk of falls. *Neurology* **2013**, *81*, 437–443. [CrossRef] [PubMed]
156. Mesbah, N.; Perry, M.; Hill, K.D.; Kaur, M.; Hale, L. Postural Stability in Older Adults With Alzheimer Disease. *Phys. Ther.* **2017**, *97*, 290–309. [CrossRef]
157. Gietzelt, M.; Wolf, K.-H.; Kohlmann, M.; Marschollek, M.; Haux, R. Measurement of Accelerometry-based Gait Parameters in People with and without Dementia in the Field. *Methods Inf. Med.* **2013**, *52*, 319–325.
158. Mc Ardle, R.; Morris, R.; Hickey, A.; Del Din, S.; Koychev, I.; Gunn, R.N.; Lawson, J.; Zamboni, G.; Ridha, B.; Sahakian, B.J.; et al. Gait in Mild Alzheimer's Disease: Feasibility of Multi-Center Measurement in the Clinic and Home with Body-Worn Sensors: A Pilot Study. *J. Alzheimers Dis.* **2018**, *63*, 331–341. [CrossRef]
159. Mirelman, A.; Gurevich, T.; Giladi, N.; Bar-Shira, A.; Orr-Urtreger, A.; Hausdorff, J.M. Gait alterations in healthy carriers of the LRRK2 G2019S mutation. *Ann. Neurol.* **2011**, *69*, 193–197. [CrossRef]
160. Phinyomark, A.; Petri, G.; Ibáñez-Marcelo, E.; Osis, S.T.; Ferber, R. Analysis of big data in gait biomechanics: Current trends and future directions. *J. Med. Biol. Eng.* **2018**, *38*, 244–260. [CrossRef]
161. Gao, C.; Sun, H.; Wang, T.; Tang, M.; Bohnen, N.I.; Müller, M.L.T.M.; Herman, T.; Giladi, N.; Kalinin, A.; Spino, C. Model-based and Model-free Machine Learning Techniques for Diagnostic Prediction and Classification of Clinical Outcomes in Parkinson's Disease. *Sci. Rep.* **2018**, *8*, 7129. [CrossRef] [PubMed]
162. Caramia, C.; Bernabucci, I.; D'Anna, C.; De Marchis, C.; Schmid, M. Gait parameters are differently affected by concurrent smartphone-based activities with scaled levels of cognitive effort. *PLoS ONE* **2017**, *12*, e0185825. [CrossRef] [PubMed]
163. Raknim, P.; Lan, K.C. Gait Monitoring for Early Neurological Disorder Detection Using Sensors in a Smartphone: Validation and a Case Study of Parkinsonism. *Telemed. E-Health* **2016**, *22*, 75–81. [CrossRef] [PubMed]
164. LeMoyne, R.; Heerinckx, F.; Aranca, T.; De Jager, R.; Zesiewicz, T.; Saal, H.J. Wearable body and wireless inertial sensors for machine learning classification of gait for people with Friedreich's ataxia. In Proceedings of the 13th Annual Body Sensor Networks Conference, BSN 2016, San Francisco, CA, USA, 14–17 June 2016; Institute of Electrical and Electronics Engineers Inc.: Piscataway, NJ, USA, 2016; pp. 147–151.
165. Costa, L.; Gago, M.F.; Yelshyna, D.; Ferreira, J.; Silva, H.D.; Rocha, L.; Sousa, N.; Bicho, E. Application of Machine Learning in Postural Control Kinematics for the Diagnosis of Alzheimer's Disease. *Comput. Intell. Neurosci.* **2016**, *3891253*. [CrossRef] [PubMed]

166. Duda, R.O.; Hart, P.E.; Stork, D.G. *Pattern classification*; John Wiley & Sons, 2012; ISBN 111858600X.
167. Abdulhay, E.; Arunkumar, N.; Narasimhan, K.; Vellaiappan, E.; Venkatraman, V. Gait and tremor investigation using machine learning techniques for the diagnosis of Parkinson disease. *Futur. Gener. Comput. Syst.* **2018**, *83*, 366–373. [CrossRef]
168. Aich, S.; Choi, K.; Park, J.; Kim, H.C.; Seoul National, U. Prediction of Parkinson disease using nonlinear classifiers with decision tree using gait dynamics. In Proceedings of the 4th International Conference on Biomedical and Bioinformatics Engineering, ICBBE 2017, Seoul, Korea, 12–14 November 2017; Association for Computing Machinery: New York, NY, USA, 2017; Volume Part F1338, pp. 52–57.
169. Cuzzolin, F.; Sapienza, M.; Esser, P.; Saha, S.; Franssen, M.M.; Collett, J.; Dawes, H. Metric learning for Parkinsonian identification from IMU gait measurements. *Gait Posture* **2017**, *54*, 127–132. [CrossRef]
170. Mannini, A.; Trojaniello, D.; Cereatti, A.; Sabatini, A.M. A machine learning framework for gait classification using inertial sensors: Application to elderly, post-stroke and huntington's disease patients. *Sensors* **2016**, *16*, 134. [CrossRef]
171. Papavasileiou, I.; Zhang, W.; Wang, X.; Bi, J.; Zhang, L.; Han, S. Classification of Neurological Gait Disorders Using Multi-task Feature Learning. In Proceedings of the 2nd IEEE International Conference on Connected Health: Applications, Systems and Engineering Technologies, CHASE 2017, Philadelphia, PA, USA, 17–19 July 2017; Institute of Electrical and Electronics Engineers Inc.: Piscataway, NJ, USA, 2017; pp. 195–204.
172. Ceseracciu, E.; Sawacha, Z.; Cobelli, C. Comparison of markerless and marker-based motion capture technologies through simultaneous data collection during gait: Proof of concept. *PLoS ONE* **2014**, *9*, e87640. [CrossRef]
173. Schmitz, A.; Ye, M.; Shapiro, R.; Yang, R.; Noehren, B. Accuracy and repeatability of joint angles measured using a single camera markerless motion capture system. *J. Biomech.* **2014**, *47*, 587–591. [CrossRef]
174. Müller, B.; Ilg, W.; Giese, M.A.; Ludolph, N. Validation of enhanced kinect sensor based motion capturing for gait assessment. *PLoS ONE* **2017**, *12*, e0175813. [CrossRef]
175. Dekhtyar, S.; Wang, H.-X.; Scott, K.; Goodman, A.; Koupil, I.; Herlitz, A. A life-course study of cognitive reserve in dementia—From childhood to old age. *Am. J. Geriatr. Psychiatry* **2015**, *23*, 885–896. [CrossRef] [PubMed]

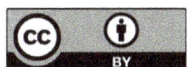

© 2019 by the authors. Licensee MDPI, Basel, Switzerland. This article is an open access article distributed under the terms and conditions of the Creative Commons Attribution (CC BY) license (http://creativecommons.org/licenses/by/4.0/).

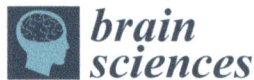

Review

Parkinsonisms and Glucocerebrosidase Deficiency: A Comprehensive Review for Molecular and Cellular Mechanism of Glucocerebrosidase Deficiency

Emilia M. Gatto [1,*], Gustavo Da Prat [1], Jose Luis Etcheverry [1], Guillermo Drelichman [2] and Martin Cesarini [1]

[1] Department of Neurology, Parkinson's Disease and Movement Disorders Section, Institute of Neuroscience of Buenos Aires (INEBA), Guardia Vieja 4435, Buenos Aires C1192AAW, Argentina; gustavoda_prat@hotmail.com (G.D.P.); jletcheverry_1@yahoo.com.ar (G.L.E.); martincesarini23@gmail.com (M.C.)

[2] Hospital de Niños Ricardo Gutiérrez, Gallo 1330, Buenos Aires C1425EFD, Argentina; drgdrelichman@yahoo.com.ar

[*] Correspondence: emiliamgatto@gmail.com; Tel./Fax: +54-11-4954-7070 (ext. 294)

Received: 2 January 2019; Accepted: 30 January 2019; Published: 1 February 2019

Abstract: In the last years, lysosomal storage diseases appear as a bridge of knowledge between rare genetic inborn metabolic disorders and neurodegenerative diseases such as Parkinson's disease (PD) or frontotemporal dementia. Epidemiological studies helped promote research in the field that continues to improve our understanding of the link between mutations in the glucocerebrosidase (*GBA*) gene and PD. We conducted a review of this link, highlighting the association in *GBA* mutation carriers and in Gaucher disease type 1 patients (GD type 1). A comprehensive review of the literature from January 2008 to December 2018 was undertaken. Relevance findings include: (1) There is a bidirectional interaction between GBA and α- synuclein in protein homeostasis regulatory pathways involving the clearance of aggregated proteins. (2) The link between GBA deficiency and PD appears not to be restricted to α–synuclein aggregates but also involves *Parkin* and *PINK1* mutations. (3) Other factors help explain this association, including early and later endosomes and the lysosomal-associated membrane protein 2A (LAMP-2A) involved in the chaperone-mediated autophagy (CMA). (4) The best knowledge allows researchers to explore new therapeutic pathways alongside substrate reduction or enzyme replacement therapies.

Keywords: glucocerebrosidase; Parkinson's disease; Gaucher disease

---

1. Introduction

In the past decade, advances in the knowledge of the pathophysiological process of Parkinson's disease (PD) have shed light on the comprehensive mechanisms involved in protein accumulation and aggregation in neurodegenerative diseases [1–3].

Parkinson's is the second most common neurodegenerative disorder. Criteria for diagnosis were redefined in 2015 by Postuma et al., with multiple genes identified as causative or as an increased risk factor [2].

In PD, a complex underlying physiopathology involving molecular processes results in alpha synuclein (α-syn) misfolding, leading abnormal aggregation and the accumulation of insoluble α-syn.

A key player in this matter is the lysosomal-autophagy system (LAS), being an important target for many new therapeutic targets in current clinical trials [1].

New genetic findings help support a concomitant dysfunctional proteostasis involving several systems, including the ubiquitin–proteasome system (UPS), chaperones, and the LAS [1,4,5].

The major candidate gene involved in PD with autosomal dominant inheritance are leucine-rich repeat kinase 2 (*LRRK2*), alpha-synuclein (*SNCA*), vacuolar sorting protein 35 (*VPS35*), and DnaJ homolog subfamily C member 13 (*DNAJC13*). In the recessive pattern the major genes players are *Parkin*, *PINK1*, and *DJ1*, as well as *GBA* [6–8].

Although the understanding of these gene functions is incomplete, several of them are involved in different protein and organelle clearance pathways.

In this sense, the homeostasis of α-synuclein depends on the ubiquitin–proteasome system (UBQ-PS) and the LAS that comprise the chaperone-mediated autophagy and macroautophagy [9]. The *SNCA* mutations and multiplications promote the accumulation of α-synuclein oligomers inhibiting the UBQ-PS and macroautophagy.

The *LRRK2* gene encodes a kinase with a protein–protein interaction, involved in transcription, translation, or apoptotic processes, and in membrane trafficking and cytoskeletal function [10]. The *LRRK2* and *G2019S* mutations have been reported to be associated with LAS and mitochondrial impairments probably mediated by a gain-of-function effect.

In the same way, deficiency and mutations in VPS35 (the encoded protein is involved in the retromer complex) not only act in the recycling of membrane proteins via retrograde transport from endosomes back to the trans-Golgi (endosome-to-Golgi retrieval) but also have been associated with decreased cellular levels of the lysosome-associated membrane glycoprotein 2A (LAMP-2A), a protein membrane involved in lysosome translocation, affecting once again the LAS [11].

Among the recessive genes linked to PD, proteins encoded by *PARK2* and *PINK1* cooperate in the clearance of damaged mitochondria through mitophagy. Impaired degradation of MIRO (a protein in the outer mitochondrial membrane that connects the organelle to microtubule motors) seems to have a role in defective clearance of damaged mitochondria [6–8].

Parkin is an E3 ubiquitin ligase protein, catalyzing the transfer of ubiquitin to its specific target protein; PINK1 is a mitochondrial kinase that localizes to damaged mitochondria and recruits Parkin in the outer mitochondrial membrane to initiate polyubiquitination of mitofusins for fusion and fission of damaged mitochondria or clearance by UBQ-PS or autophagy involving, again, the LAS [12].

Inborn errors of metabolism (IEM) are characterized by mutations in genes coding enzymes involved in different metabolic pathways. Lysosomal diseases enclose an extensive number of genetic disorders characterized by malfunction of the lysosomal enzymes in the LAS [13,14].

Gaucher disease (GD) is the most frequent lysosomal storage disease inherited in an autosomal recessive pattern [4,15,16]. More than 300 different mutations of the glucocerebrosidase 1 (GBA1) gene have been described, with over 12 different genotypes. This gene is located on chromosome 1q2 and encodes glucocerebrosidase (GCase). The GCase enzyme catalyzes the hydrolysis of glycolipid glucocerebroside to ceramide and glucose [17]. It is synthesized in the endoplasmic reticulum (ER) and transported to lysosomes via lysosomal membrane protein 2 (LIMP2). The binding of GCase to LIMP2 is facilitated by the neutral pH of the ER. These proteins remain together at the Golgi apparatus and endosomes, but their dissociation is facilitated by acidic pH into the lysosome [18,19].

Glucocerebroside accumulation results in a systemic disease with distinctive phenotypes [4]. The clinical classification describes three different subtypes, GD 1, 2, and 3, respectively [13,20].

Type 2 or acute neuronopathic is the more severe phenotype and is beyond the scope of the present review, affecting perinatal and infancy with a severe prognosis and limited survival of no more than 3 years, with severe ocular abnormalities, development delay and brainstem involvement and severe hematological and visceral compromise.

Gaucher disease type 3 is called subacute neuronopathic variant with age at onset in childhood with neurological involvement including oculomotor abnormalities, ataxia, seizures (myoclonic epilepsy) and dementia.

Finally, GD type 1 is classically mentioned as non-neuronopathic, with a wide spectrum of age at onset, anemia, thrombocytopenia, and enlargement of the spleen, skeletal abnormalities, interstitial disease and pulmonary hypertension. However, it has been estimated that a neurological symptom occurs in 50% of patients with GD1, and it is possible to identify a neurological abnormality during examination in 30% of patients without neurological complaints [21–23].

Epidemiological studies in GD type 1 showed an association between GCase deficiency and Parkinsonism. In fact, the homozygous and heterozygous mutations, constitute a strongest risk factor for the development of PD and Lewy Body Dementia (LBP) [4].

This review primarily focuses on the potential link between GCase deficiency and PD and identifies new potential common pharmacological approaches to GD, a rare treatable disorder, and PD [24].

2. Methods

2.1. Search Strategy and Selection Criteria

A literature search was conducted to identify relevant articles published in English, based on Medline (via Pubmed) from January 2008 to December 2018. One local article in Spanish was included [25].

2.2. Lysosomal Diseases and Gaucher Epidemiology

Several movement disorders have been described in the spectrum of lysosomal diseases, among them levodopa responsive parkinsonism and parkinsonism plus (ataxia, dystonia or spasticity) [4,13,21,26]. In this sense, *GBA* mutation, neuronal ceroid lipofuscinosis, Kufor–Rakeb disease, Niemann Pick type C are among the lysosomal disorders associated to hypokinetic movement disorders and more specifically to Parkinsonisms [21].

In a recent study of a cohort of 76 individuals with different lysosomal diseases, GD was identified in 3.99% of them [26].

Among the conferred risk of genes and genetic loci associated with the development of idiopathic PD, it was observed that *GBA* mutations are the most common genetic risk factor for developing PD [27,28]. Furthermore, GD patients and GBA mutation carriers are at higher risk of developing parkinsonism. Large epidemiological studies found that *GBA* mutations were significantly prevalent in PD patients (Odd Ratio: 5.43); between 5% and 20% of all PD patients have a *GBA* mutation [4,29–31].

Further, *GBA1* mutations are the most common genetic risk factor for developing PD [27]. The worldwide range of prevalence of GD type 1 has been estimated at between 1:40,000 and 1:60,000, with the highest prevalence in Ashkenazi Jews (1:850) [32] (19.20%), intermediated prevalence in the North American population (12.93%–15.90%), and lowest in the Asian population (2.70%–3.70%) [27,33–46]. This association is stronger for dementia with Lewy bodies (LBD).

Epidemiological data suggest that non-neuropathic GD type 1 needs to be redefined, taking into account the occurrence of neurological signs and symptoms such as movement disorders, cognitive decline, slow saccades and progressive supranuclear palsy [21,47].

2.3. Phenotype/Genotype: Clinical Features

From a clinical point of view, some differences arise between idiopathic PD and *GBA* mutated carriers (*GBA*mtt carriers) with PD. For instance, PD-GBA carriers tend to have a younger age at onset. A good response to l-dopa is a common finding; however, there is contrasting evidence for the occurrence of levodopa-induced dyskinesias, and in those cases the risk is related to the age at onset.

Non-motor symptoms, autonomic dysfunction (including enteric, sexual and urinary dysfunctions as well as orthostatic hypotension), fatigue, anxiety, pain, REM behavior disorders (RBD) and cognitive impairment are more frequent in *GBA*mtt carriers than in individuals with idiopathic Parkinsonism.

A multi-domain impairment has been reported involving memory, visuospatial, abstraction, orientation, working memory, executive, visuospatial abilities and visual short-term memory.

Mood, behavioral and psychiatric symptoms appear as a common manifestation in *GBA*-PD, with earlier development of psychosis and hallucinations, as well as higher prevalence of depression, apathy and anxiety [4,48].

2.4. Biomarkers

Clinical and neuroimaging biomarkers in *GBA*mtt carriers with PD with respect to the idiopathic PD (iPD) patients are presented in Table 1.

Table 1. Clinical and neuroimaging potential biomarkers of Gaucher disease (GD) type 1.

Biomarker	Observation	References
Clinical biomarker	Early multidomain cognitive impairment. More severe Levodopa induced dyskinesias.	
Transcranial sonography	Nigral hyperechogenicity.	[49]
PET 1 8F dopa	Decreased striatal dopamine synthesis, similar to iPD. Bilateral asymmetric reduction in striatal uptake.	[50,51]
fMRI	Significant hypometabolism in glucose metabolism in supplementary motor area and parieto-occipital cortices. Hypermetabolism of the lentiform nuclei and thalamus. Decrease in the parieto-occipital and to a certain degree anteromedial frontal cortex.	[52]
Diffusion tensor MRI	Decreased frontal cortico-cortical and parahippocampal tracts in GBA-PD. Decreased fractional anisotropy of the corpus callosum, olfactory tract, anterior limb of the internal capsule, cingulum, external capsule bilaterally, and left superior longitudinal fasciculus.	[52]
Postsynaptic DA 11 C-Raclopride	Postsynaptic dopamine terminal persistence of higher putaminal uptake in advanced disease.	[53]

GD: Gaucher Disease. PET: Positron Emission Tomography. GD-PD: Gaucher Disease–Parkinson Disease. iPD: idiopathic Parkinson Disease. fMRI: functional magnetic resonance imaging. MRI: magnetic resonance imaging. DA: dopamine.

2.4.1. Wet Biomarkers in GBA Mutation Carriers PD

Dried blood spot and cerebrospinal fluid (CSF) studies demonstrated a decreased glucocerebrosidase (GCase) activity in PD patients with and without GBA mutation carriers versus healthy controls. The decreased activity correlates with a worse cognitive performance [54–56].

2.4.2. Prodromal Signs in PD-GBA Patients

As in iPD, prodromal signs have been described in GD type 1 patients and *GBA* mtt carriers. Hyposmia, cognitive dysfunction (involvement of attention, working memory and speed of memory), subtle motor signs, depression, smell and autonomic dysfunction were more common in GBA patients and carriers. Thus, these are suggested as potential neurodegeneration markers in GD patients and carriers [35,47].

Gatto et al. conducted a study in the city of Buenos Aires, Argentina where prodromal clinical markers of PD were explored in GD patients [57]. A total of 26 patients with GD1 were included, and all of them were under enzymatic replacement therapy. Questionnaires used to identify non-motor PD symptoms revealed that 26.9% had parasomnias, 7.69% RBD and constipation, 3.84% hyposmia and 11.53% depression. Some 44.4% had some degree of cognitive impairment. Although none of the patients studied fulfilled Queen Square Brain Bank criteria for PD, the presence of non-motor symptoms, as in other series, could be used as potential prodromic biomarkers for Parkinsonism [57].

2.4.3. Cognition in GBA Homozygous and Heterozygous GBA Mutations Carriers

Although data on cognition in asymptomatic *GBA* mutation carriers are scarce, several authors found substantially increased risk of conversion to dementia in GBA mutations carriers [58].

GD type1 and GBA mtt carriers were associated with an earlier age at onset of PD and a higher MDS-UPDRS III, associated with attention, working memory and speed memory impairment. In these cases, the cognitive decline represents one of the most debilitating manifestation impairing the quality of life [59]).

Genetic factors could contribute to modulate the risk of PD and dementia in *GBA* carriers. For instance, null/severe L444P mutations have the highest risk, while an intermediate risk has been reported for mild mutations such as N370S, and the lowest risk was associated with a E326K polymorphism.

In a study conducted by Mata et al. in 2016 [60], the authors found that pathogenic mutations and the E326K polymorphism within the *GBA* gene were associated with a higher prevalence of dementia involving working memory/executive function and visuospatial abilities. These results suggest that even homozygous carriers for E326K polymorphism do not develop GD; this single nucleotide polymorphism might influence the risk of PD cognitive dysfunction.

Controversial results were reported when the *LRRK2* and *GBA* gene mutation carrier cohorts were compared. Some authors failed to identify any cognitive difference in asymptomatic *GBA* and *LRRK2* mutation carriers [61], whereas others identified a lower mean MoCA score and a worsening verbal memory in non-manifesting *LRRK2* carriers with respect to the *GBA* mutations carriers [62]. It remains under discussion whether a more diffuse and extensive neocortical Lewy body pathology increases the risk of cognitive dysfunction in homozygous and heterozygous *GBA* mtt carriers. However, only a marginal difference was found in a PD clinic pathological study performed in *GBA* mutation carriers and non-carriers.

Finally, as in iPD, depression in *GBA* carriers appears as a prodromal factor influencing the performance in cognitive testing.

2.4.4. The Role of Autophagy in Lysosomal Diseases and Neurodegeneration (α-synuclein)

An extensive number of experimental studies showed that *GBA* can stabilize α-synuclein oligomers which in turn inhibit *GBA* function, causing glycocylceramide (GlcCer) accumulation and further attenuate α-synuclein aggregation [63].

Under normal conditions, the autophagy system allows the cell to degrade different compounds. The different types of autophagy are: Microautophagy, macroautophagy and chaperone-mediated autophagy (CMA). These are carried out differently, but the final common pathway is the lysosome, a key player in proteins, lipids and organelles degradation [64,65].

We make a special note of alpha synuclein (α-syn), α-syn is a presynaptic protein, involved in neurotransmitter release through the SNARE complex. When an impairment in the degradation of α-syn occurs, this protein accumulates as insoluble fibrils, giving rise to toxicity in multiple cellular processes (lysosome, mitochondria, proteasome and cellular membrane recycle) [66,67].

It is thought that this accumulation is derived from Lewy body pathology. However, some authors propose a protective cycle through protein accumulation mediated by α-syn. Interestingly, α-syn accumulation leads to reduced GCase and GCase accumulation makes the cell prone to α-syn deposition. Thus, this pathological cycle between GCase and α-syn worsens the condition [4,29].

Cellular protein accumulation promotes what is known as endoplasmic reticulum stress (ERS). When activated, it leads to an apoptotic pathway. Moreover, when ERS is activated there is an inhibition of other ER substrates as well as malfunction of Golgi traffic. This process has also been observed in PD patients with *PARK2* mutations, thus suggesting that ERS has a role in PD pathology [4,29].

2.4.5. *GBA* Gene Mutations

Next-generation sequencing technologies have had a dramatic impact on the field of genomic research and on knowledge of *GBA* mutations. This autosomal recessive disease is caused by different mutations in the *GBA* gene that encode lysosomal enzyme glucocerebrosidase (Gcase), (in chromosome 1q21 [68]). This gene contains 11 exons and 10 introns, covering 7.6 kilobases (kb) of sequence. Over 300 mutations, including point mutations, insertions, deletions and frameshift mutations, in the *GBA* gene have been identified; seven of them account for approximately 96% of the mutant alleles in Ashkenazi Jews (AJ). The most common mutations are: K198T, E326K, T369M, N370S, V394L, D409H, L444P, and R496H. Both N370S and R496H are considered mild mutations, whereas E326K, N370S, and L444P are associated with severe neuronopathic forms of GD. The most deleterious is considered to be L44P, causing high protein destabilization, related to its position at the beginning of the beta sheet [4,16,68,69].

The most common mutation in the *GBA* gene worldwide is N370S/N370S, followed by N370S/L444P [70]. Severe *GBA* mutations (L444P) cause neuronopathic GD onset during infancy and childhood, rapid progression, severe neurological symptoms and shorter life expectancy. Mild GD is caused by N370S mutations; interestingly over 50% of GD-PD are homozygous for these mutations, and 90% of these patients carry at least one N370S mutation. This is important to take into consideration for carriers of *GBA* mutations where severe mutations are related to a higher risk of developing PD7. Moreover, mutations in *GBA* coding for pathogenic neuropathic GD and heterozygous severe forms accelerate cognitive decline in these patients [71].

The increased PD risk in *GBA* mutation carriers is racially dependent. The analysis in AJ population identified 84 insGG and R496H variants as the exclusive risk for increased PD in this population, whereas, in non-AJ, L444P, R120W, IVS2+1G > A, H255Q, D409H, RecNciI, E326K, and T369M represent the highest risk variants with an ethnic distribution. The N370S appears as a risk variant of PD in AJ and non-AJ populations, while L444P increased the risk of PD in all groups in non-AJ ethnicity [72]. Other variants, including N370S, H255Q, D409H and E326K, exclusively increased PD risk in non-AJ European/West Asians, whereas R120W increased PD risk in East Asians.

The polymorphic variant E326K represents an interesting variant to analyze, taking into account that controversial results have been reported regarding the risk of PD. A recent meta-analysis reveals that E326K of *GBA* is associated with a risk of PD in total populations, Asians and Caucasians [73,74].

In the Argentinean GD population, the prevalent variants were: Genotype N307S/other allele (82.5%), N307S/L444P and N307S/N307S [25].

A correlation genotype/phenotype is presented in Table 2.

Table 2. Phenotype/genotype correlation.

	Null or Severe GBAmtt	Mild GD
	L444P	N307S
Phenotype	Onset infancy and childhood, rapid progression shorter life expectancy, and appearance of more severe neurologic features (GD2, GD3)	50% GD-PD homozygous for N307S 90% GD-PD carry at least one N307S mutation

For *GBA* mutation carriers, "severe" mutations have a higher risk of Parkinson's disease (PD) than "mild mutations," as well as early age onset of symptoms, initial bradykinesia and family history of dementia [14,62]. GD: Gaucher disease. *GBA*: glucocerebrosidase. GD-PD: Gaucher-DiseaseParkinson Disease.

2.5. *Gaucher and PD: the Ethiopatogenic Link*

Parkinson's disease is the second most common neurodegenerative disorder worldwide. Multiple pathways for cortical and subcortical structures are involved in the pathology. The hallmark for PD is the intracellular aggregation of α-synuclein. As discussed earlier, PD emerges as a consequence of the failure of multiple cellular pathways to avoid damage by toxic protein accumulation. The failure of protein homeostasis leads to dysfunction of the two major catabolic pathways, UPS, and the autophagy-lysosomal pathway (ALP), as well as mitochondrial, ER and vesicular transport [75,76].

Alpha-synuclein constitutes the major component of LB. It has been proposed that LB deposition follows a sequential pattern of accumulation, as proposed by Braak et al. in 2003 [77]. Initially affecting the dorsal nucleus of the glossopharyngeal and vagal nerves, brainstem, mesocortex and lastly neocortex [4].

Early studies demonstrated a colocalization of mutant GCase in LB and Lewy neuritis (LN) in subjects carrying *GBA*.

Moreover, several recent studies have shown that the levels of GCase catalytic activity is reduced in *GBA* homozygous and heterozygous carriers as well as mRNA GCase levels. The decreased GCase activity was not restricted to *GBA* carriers but was also identified in iPD and DLB, with a marked distribution in different brain areas and more pronounced in Substantia Nigra (SN) [1].

The decrease of GCase activity correlates with *GBA* post translational regulators, protein interactors, lysosomal integral membrane protein 2 (LIMP-2) and saposin C (SapC) [1].

Several GCase mutations, including N370S and L444P, unfold in the ER, activating the unfolded protein response (UPR).

Pathways of GCase from the ER to the lysosome in wild and mutant GCase are presented in Figure 1.

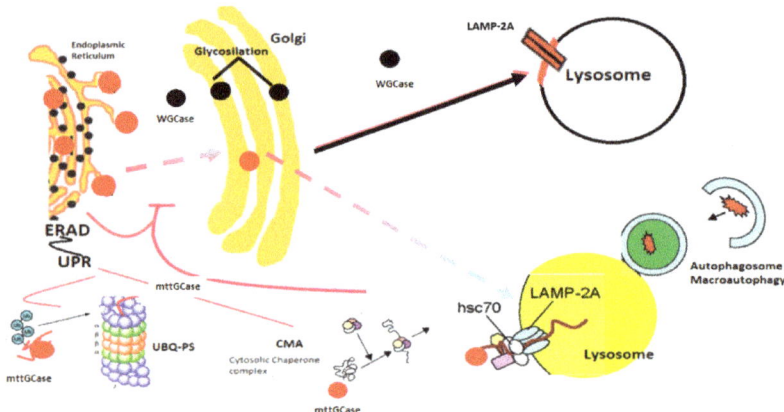

Figure 1. Glucocerebrosidase pathway: Black circles represent wild-type glucocerebrosidase (wtCGase) that is produced in the endoplasmic reticulum (ER), glycosylated in the Golgi, and is translocated to the lysosome in a LIMP-2 dependent process, where it degrades glucosylceramide substrates. Red circles represent mutant enzyme (mttGCase), not folded correctly and inducing the ER stress response. This ER stress response comprises: The ER-associated protein degradation (ERAD) that re-translocated mttGCase from the ER to the cytoplasm and unfolded protein response (UPR) in an attempt to re-establish homeostasis via ubiquitin proteasome system (UBQ-PS), cytosolic chaperone complex (CMA) represents another pathway to refold mttGCase by hsc70 linked to the LAMP-2A to deliver the protein to the lysosome. The dotted line represents the small fraction of mttGCase that could take the normal pathway.

Mutant GCase (mtt GCase) leads to ER stress (ERAD), inducement of UPR, proteosomal breakdown by UBQ-PS, cytoplasmic chaperone-mediated autophagy (CMA), delivery of unfolded proteins into the lysosome by chaperones, and the involvement of LAMP-2A, a protein membrane, in translocation. Glycocylceramide accumulates in the lysosome. Macroautophagy is involved in the degradation of damaged organelles and aggregated proteins and modified lipids [78].

The GCase needs to interact at the ER with LIMP-2 to be glycosylated and transported to lysosome to exert hydrolytic activity on GlcCer [79].

2.6. α-Synuclein and GCase Link

The PD pathophysiologic mechanisms are very complex, involving several pathways related to a failure of α-synuclein degradation, oxidative stress, neuroinflammation, and mitochondrial and synaptic dysfunction. Ubiquitin proteasome dysfunction, macroautophagy and CMA impairment promote α-synuclein aggregation and a prion-like transmission.

Both PD and GD share pathological processes that result in lysosomal dysfunction, dysfunctional lipid metabolism, prion-like transmission and bidirectional feedback loop. As a result of the incomplete clearance of these substrates, in GBA-PD, a decrease in GCase activity results in increased levels of glucosylceramide, affecting autophagy and promoting α-synuclein accumulation by stabilization of α-synuclein oligomeric forms [80]. High levels of intracellular α-synuclein prones subsequent ERAD and contributes to GCase glycosylation as well as trafficking dysfunction from ER to Golgi and finally to lysosomes. This pathological loop enhances, so accumulation of glucosylceramide causes α-synuclein, and high α-synuclein levels inhibit GCase. The final consequence is a loss of lysosomal activity and neuronal death [4,81].

Recently, Thomas et al. [82] identified a membrane lipid composition alteration in Drosophila mutants with deletions in the *GBA* ortholog Gba1b. This membrane alteration increases the formation and release of extracellular vesicles that might lead to aggregates seeding and spread cell-to-cell neurodegeneration as a major mechanism for the association of *GBA* and PD neurodegeneration.

2.7. Parkin-Pink1 Mitochondria and GCase

Dysfunctional mitochondria and failure in mitophagy (macroautophagy) have been identified in brain tissues from GBA-PD patients and *GBA*L444P.

Furthermore, *SNCA*, *PINK1* and *PRKN*, *PARK7* and *LRRK2* have a role in the equilibrium between mitochondrial fusion and fission [83–89].

Li et al. reported, in an experimental model of GBA-PD, two mechanisms affecting mitochondria: (a) The impairment of autophagy secondary to lysosomal accumulation of glucosylceramide with decreased GBA activity, and (b) mitochondrial priming, with decreased mitochondrial fission [88,90].

The mitochondrial priming represents the *PINK1-PARK2* pathway required for the balance between fusion and fission [88].

The interaction between Parkin2 and GBA is restricted not only to mitochondrial involvement but also by competitive ubiquitination of mutant GCase, promoting protein accumulation, leading ERAD, increasing cytosolic Ca^{2+} and apoptosis [89].

2.8. Therapeutic Implications

Amongst the treatment strategies in patients with GD, either substrate reduction therapy (SRT) or enzyme replacement therapy (ERT) is traditionally employed. For the former, the target is to inhibit glucosylceramide synthase.

When considering ERT, imiglucerase (effective for GD1 patients), velaglucerase alfa and taliglucerase alfa are the available options. None of these is able to cross the blood–brain barrier (BBB), being ineffective in neurological symptoms [4].

Substrate reduction therapy is considered second in line for the treatment of GD, because of its adverse events. Some drugs are able to cross the BBB, such as miglustat, a small iminosugar with reversible inhibitor activity. It was thought that it could be useful for GD3 patients; however, a randomized study did not prove significant difference in the patients in terms of neurological symptoms [4,91].

Due to the relationship between GCase and α-synuclein deposition, new promising therapies are under investigation for patients with PD and GBA mutations. In this matter, the MOVES-PD trial has been announced, in which GZ/SAR402671 will be tested in PD patients with a single GBA mutation in order to reduce the production of glycosphingolipids [92]. On this point, Sardi et al. [93]

showed, in experimental models, that α-syn accumulation could be reduced using a glycosylceramide synthase inhibitor (GCC) called Venglustat. It was demonstrated that GCC could reduce the levels of glycosylceramide in the central nervous system (CNS), reduce the accumulation of α-syn in the hippocampus and ameliorate cognitive deficits, making this a promising disease-modifying therapy.

2.9. Future Therapies for GD

Due to the multiple cellular pathways involved in GD, other therapies that target different sites of these pathways are under investigation. Chaperones are small molecules that facilitate the correct folding and translocation of GCase, hence making them a suitable option for treating lysosomal disorders. An example of this is ambroxol (ABX).

Chaperones bind to misfolded GCase and cross BBB. Ambroxol acts as a pharmacological chaperone, enhancing lysosomal function and autophagy. It has been shown that ABX significantly increases glycosylceramidase and reduces α-syn, especially in the striatum. Antioxidative functions of ABX have also been postulated as an important property [29,94]. A novel non-inhibitory GCase chaperone, NCGC607, restored the levels of GCase activity and reduced α-syn levels in dopaminergic neurons [95].

Other therapies included histone deacetylase inhibitor, promoting the activity of the mutant GCase [96]. Also, lentiviral vectors with cellular promoters may play a role in future clinical gene therapy protocols for GD1 [96]. Autophagy enhancement through the mTor-pathway, using rapamycins, has been shown to reduce α-synuclein aggregation [4].

Recently, Zunke et al. [97] demonstrated that accumulation of glycosphingolipids in GD promote conformational changes in α-synuclein-leading aggregation and toxicity. In this scenario the reduction of glycosphingolipids appears as a potential new therapeutic pathway, taking into account the fact that this reduction was able to reduce pathology and reverse α-synuclein to the normal conformation in carrier and non-carrier PD patients.

More recently, Kim et al. [98] suggested a new therapeutic approach by inhibition of acid ceramidase. This inhibition helps increase the ceramide levels in lysosome in GCase mutant cells and reduce α-synuclein accumulation.

3. Conclusions

As previously mentioned, *GBA* mutations are the most common genetic risk factors associated with PD, especially common in AJ populations. Multiple cellular pathways are linked to GD. This includes lysosomal dysfunction, ERS, autophagy and α-syn deposition, each of them enhancing a vicious cycle of more protein misfolding and deposition. As proposed by Espay et al. [99]. Parkinson's disease could be considered as a group of disorders that share nigral dopamine-neuron degeneration; hence, PD is divided into different subgroups of PD with their own distinctive biology. This could be useful in the development of disease-modifying therapies for each subgroup of targeted patients. Parkinson's disease in GD patients could be a subgroup of patients for whom disease-modifying therapies that reduce α-syn and slow, reduce or even stop disease progression could be effective. More clinical trials are required in order to analyze these patients.

Author Contributions: E.M.G., study concept and design. G.D.P., acquisition of data. M.C., analysis and interpretation of data. J.L.E., analysis and interpretation of data. G.D., analysis of data and critical review.

Funding: This research received no external funding.

Acknowledgments: The authors would like to thank Alisdair McNeill, MRCP (UK) DCH for his critical comments and helpful suggestions; Virginia Parisi and Gabriel Persi for their scientific suggestions; and Paula Bagalio for her English review. We would also like to thank patients and their families.

Conflicts of Interest: Emilia M. Gatto received honoraria as speaker by Sanofi-Genzyme. Sanofi-Genzyme had no role in the design, execution, interpretation, or writing of the study. Gustavo Da Prat had no conflict of interest. Martin Cesarini received honoraria as speaker by Sanofi-Genzyme. Sanofi-Genzyme had no role in the design, execution, interpretation, or writing of the study. Jose Luis Etcheverry received honoraria as speaker by

Sanofi-Genzyme. Sanofi-Genzyme had no role in the design, execution, interpretation, or writing of the study. Guillermo Drelichman received honoraria as speaker and external advisor by Sanofi-Genzyme. Sanofi-Genzyme had no role in the design, execution, interpretation, or writing of the study.

References

1. Moors, T.E.; Paciotti, S.; Ingrassia, A.; Quadri, M.; Breedveld, G.; Tasegian, A.; Chiasserini, D.; Eusebi, P.; Duran-Pacheco, G.; Kremer, T.; et al. Characterization of Brain Lysosomal Activities in GBA-Related and Sporadic Parkinson's Disease and Dementia with Lewy Bodies. *Mol. Neurobiol.* **2018**, 1–12. [CrossRef] [PubMed]
2. Postuma, R.B.; Berg, D.; Stern, M.; Poewe, W.; Olanow, C.W.; Oertel, W.; Obeso, J.; Marek, K.; Litvan, I.; Lang, A.E.; et al. MDS clinical diagnostic criteria for Parkinson's disease. *Mov. Disord.* **2015**, *12*, 1591–1601. [CrossRef] [PubMed]
3. Thibaudeau, T.A.; Anderson, R.T.; Smith, D.M. A common mechanism of proteasome impairment by neurodegenerative disease-associated oligomers. *Nat. Commun.* **2018**, *9*, 1097. [CrossRef] [PubMed]
4. Balestrino, R.; Schapira, A. Glucocerebrosidase and Parkinson Disease: Molecular, Clinical and Therapeutic Implications. *Neuroscientist* **2018**, *5*, 540–559. [CrossRef] [PubMed]
5. Li, S.; Le, W. Milestones of Parkinson's Disease Research: 200 Years of History and Beyond. *Neurosci. Bull.* **2017**, *33*, 598–602. [CrossRef] [PubMed]
6. Kim, C.Y.; Alcalay, R.N. Genetic Forms of Parkinson's Disease. *Semin. Neurol.* **2017**, *37*, 135–146. [CrossRef] [PubMed]
7. Domingo, A.; Klein, C. Genetics of Parkinson disease. *Handb. Clin. Neurol.* **2018**, *147*, 211–227. [CrossRef] [PubMed]
8. Poewe, W.; Seppi, K.; Tanner, C.M.; Halliday, G.M.; Brundin, P.; Volkmann, J.; Schrag, A.E.; Lang, A.E. Parkinson disease. *Nat. Rev. Dis. Primers* **2017**, *3*, 17013. [CrossRef]
9. Xilouri, M.; Brekk, O.R.; Stefanis, L. Alpha-synuclein and protein degradation systems: A reciprocal relationship. *Mol. Neurobiol.* **2013**, *47*, 537–551. [CrossRef]
10. Kett, L.R.; Boassa, D.; Ho, C.C.; Rideout, H.J.; Hu, J.; Terada, M.; Ellisman, M.; Dauer, W.T. LRRK2 Parkinson disease mutations enhance its microtubule association. *Hum. Mol. Genet.* **2012**, *21*, 890–899. [CrossRef]
11. Harbour, M.E.; Breusegem, S.Y.A.; Antrobus, R.; Freeman, C.; Reid, E.; Seaman, M.N.J. The cargo-selective retromer complex is a recruiting hub for protein complexes that regulate endosomal tubule dynamics. *J. Cell Sci.* **2010**, *123*, 3703–3717. [CrossRef] [PubMed]
12. Deng, H.; Dodson, M.W.; Huang, H.; Guo, M. The Parkinson's disease genes pink1 and parkin promote mitochondrial fission and/or inhibit fusion in Drosophila. *Proc. Natl. Acad. Sci. USA* **2008**, *105*, 14503–14508. [CrossRef] [PubMed]
13. Ferreira, C.R.; Gahl, W.A. Lysosomal storage diseases. *Transl. Sci. Rare Dis.* **2017**, *2*, 1–71. [CrossRef] [PubMed]
14. Kielian, T. Lysosomal storage disorders: Pathology within the lysosome and beyond. *J. Neurochem.* **2019**. [CrossRef] [PubMed]
15. Kinghorn, K.J.; Asghari, A.M.; Castillo-Quan, J.I. The emerging role of autophagic-lysosomal dysfunction in Gaucher Disease and Parkinson's disease. *Neural Regen. Res.* **2017**, *12*, 380–384. [CrossRef] [PubMed]
16. Thaler, A.; Bregman, N.; Gurevich, T.; Shiner, T.; Dror, Y.; Zmira, O.; Gan-Or, Z.; Bar-Shira, A.; Gana-Weisz, M.; Orr-Urtreger, A.; et al. Parkinson's disease phenotype is influenced by the severity of the mutations in the GBA gene. *Parkinsonism Relat. Disord.* **2018**, *55*, 45–49. [CrossRef] [PubMed]
17. Beutler, E.; Gelbart, T. Mutation analysis in Gaucher disease. *Am. J. Med. Genet.* **1992**, *44*, 389–390. [CrossRef] [PubMed]
18. Reczek, D.; Schwake, M.; Schröder, J.; Hughes, H.; Blanz, J.; Jin, X.; Brondyk, W.; Van Patten, S.; Edmunds, T.; Saftig, P. LIMP-2 is a receptor for lysosomal mannose-6-phosphate-independent targeting of beta-glucocerebrosidase. *Cell* **2007**, *131*, 770–783. [CrossRef]
19. Jović, M.; Kean, M.J.; Szentpetery, Z.; Polevoy, G.; Gingras, A.C.; Brill, J.A.; Balla, T. Two phosphatidylinositol 4-kinases control lysosomal delivery of the Gaucher disease enzyme, β-glucocerebrosidase. *Mol. Biol. Cell* **2012**, *23*, 1533–1545. [CrossRef]

20. Dandana, A.; Ben Khelifa, S.; Chahed, H.; Miled, A.; Ferchichi, S. Gaucher Disease: Clinical, Biological and Therapeutic Aspects. *Pathobiology* **2016**, *83*, 13–23. [CrossRef]
21. Rodriguez-Porcel, F.; Espay, A.J.; Carecchio, M. Parkinson disease in Gaucher disease. *J. Clin. Mov. Disord.* **2017**, *4*, 7. [CrossRef] [PubMed]
22. Siebert, M.; Sidransky, E.; Westbroek, W. Glucocerebrosidase is shaking up the synucleinopathies. *Brain* **2014**, *137*, 1304–1322. [CrossRef] [PubMed]
23. Capablo Liesa, J.L.; de Cabezón, A.S.; Alarcia Alejos, R.; Ara Callizo, J.R. Clinical characteristics of the neurological forms of Gaucher's disease. *Med. Clin.* **2011**, *137* (Suppl. 1), 6–11. [CrossRef]
24. Jinnah, H.A.; Albanese, A.; Bhatia, K.P.; Cardoso, F.; Da Prat, G.; de Koning, T.J.; Espay, A.J.; Fung, V.; Garcia-Ruiz, P.J.; Gershanik, O.; et al. International Parkinson's Disease Movement Disorders Society Task Force on Rare Movement Disorders. Treatable inherited rare movement disorders. *Mov. Disord.* **2018**, *33*, 21–35. [CrossRef] [PubMed]
25. Drelichman, G.; Fernández Escobar, N.; Basack, N.; Aversa, L.; Kohan, R.; Watman, N.; Bolesina, M.; Elena, G.; Veber, S.E.; Dragosky, M.; et al. *Enfermedad de Gaucher en Argentina Un informe del Registro Internacional de Gaucher y del Grupo Argentino de Diagnóstico y Tratamiento de la Enfermedad de Gaucher 12Revista de Hematologia*; 17-Suplemento Enfermedad de Gaucher; Sociedad Argentina de Hematología HEMATOLOGÍA: Buenos Aires, Argentina, 2013; pp. 4–16.
26. Ebrahimi-Fakhari, D.; Hildebrandt, C.; Davis, P.E.; Rodan, L.H.; Anselm, I.; Bodamer, O. The Spectrum of Movement Disorders in Childhood-Onset Lysosomal Storage Diseases. *Mov. Disord. Clin. Pract.* **2018**, *5*, 149–155. [CrossRef] [PubMed]
27. Sidransky, E.; Nalls, M.A.; Aasly, J.O.; Aharon-Peretz, J.; Annesi, G.; Barbosa, E.R.; Bar-Shira, A.; Berg, D.; Bras, J.; Brice, A.; et al. Multicenter analysis of glucocerebrosidase mutations in Parkinson's disease. *N. Engl. J. Med.* **2009**, *361*, 1651–1661. [CrossRef] [PubMed]
28. Velayati, A.; Yu, W.H.; Sidransky, E. The role of glucocerebrosidase mutations in Parkinson disease and Lewy body disorders. *Curr. Neurol. Neurosci. Rep.* **2010**, *10*, 190–198. [CrossRef]
29. Gan-Or, Z.; Liong, C.; Alcalay, R.N. GBA-Associated Parkinson's Disease and Other Synucleinopathies. *Curr. Neurol. Neurosci. Rep.* **2018**, *18*, 44. [CrossRef]
30. Mitsui, J.; Mizuta, I.; Toyoda, A.; Ashida, R.; Takahashi, Y.; Goto, J.; Fukuda, Y.; Date, H.; Iwata, A.; Yamamoto, M.; et al. Mutations for Gaucher disease confer high susceptibility to Parkinson disease. *Arch. Neurol.* **2009**, *66*, 571–576. [CrossRef]
31. Alcalay, R.N.; Dinur, T.; Quinn, T.; Sakanaka, K.; Levy, O.; Waters, C.; Fahn, S.; Dorovski, T.; Chung, W.K.; Pauciulo, M.; et al. Comparison of Parkinson risk in Ashkenazi Jewish patients with Gaucher disease and GBA heterozygotes. *JAMA Neurol.* **2014**, *71*, 752–757. [CrossRef]
32. Grabowski, G.A.; Zimran, A.; Ida, H. Gaucher disease types 1 and 3: Phenotypic characterization of large populations from the ICGG Gaucher Registry. *Am. J. Hematol.* **2015**, *90*, 12–18. [CrossRef]
33. Spitz, M.; Rozenberg, R.; Pereira Lda, V.; Reis Barbosa, E. Association between Parkinson's disease and glucocerebrosidase mutations in Brazil. *Parkinsonism Relat. Disord.* **2008**, *14*, 58–62. [CrossRef] [PubMed]
34. Bultron, G.; Kacena, K.; Pearson, D.; Boxer, M.; Yang, R.; Sathe, S.; Pastores, G.; Mistry, P.K. The risk of Parkinson's disease in type 1 Gaucher disease. *J. Inherit. Metab. Dis.* **2010**, *33*, 167–173. [CrossRef] [PubMed]
35. McNeill, A.; Duran, R.; Proukakis, C.; Bras, J.; Hughes, D.; Mehta, A.; Hardy, J.; Wood, N.W.; Schapira, A.H. Hyposmia and cognitive impairment in Gaucher disease patients and carriers. *Mov. Disord.* **2012**, *27*, 526–532. [CrossRef]
36. Mao, X.; Wang, T.; Peng, R.; Chang, X.; Li, N.; Gu, Y.; Zhao, D.; Liao, Q.; Liu, M. Mutations in GBA and risk of Parkinson's disease: A meta-analysis based on 25 case-control studies. *Neurol. Res.* **2013**, *35*, 873–878. [CrossRef] [PubMed]
37. Blanz, J.; Saftig, P. Parkinson's disease: Acid-glucocerebrosidase activity and alpha-synuclein clearance. *J. Neurochem.* **2016**, *139* (Suppl. 1), 198–215. [CrossRef] [PubMed]
38. Migdalska-Richards, A.; Schapira, A.H. The relationship between glucocerebrosidase mutations and Parkinson disease. *J. Neurochem.* **2016**, *139* (Suppl. 1), 77–90. [CrossRef]
39. Aflaki, E.; Westbroek, W.; Sidransky, E. The Complicated Relationship between Gaucher Disease and Parkinsonism: Insights from a Rare Disease. *Neuron* **2017**, *93*, 737–746. [CrossRef]
40. O'Regan, G.; deSouza, R.M.; Balestrino, R.; Schapira, A.H. Glucocerebrosidase Mutations in Parkinson Disease. *J. Parkinsons Dis.* **2017**, *7*, 411–422. [CrossRef]

41. Standaert, D.G. What would Dr. James parkinson think today? Mutations in beta-glucocerebrosidase and risk of Parkinson's disease. *Mov. Disord.* **2017**, *32*, 1341–1342. [CrossRef]
42. Giraldo, P.; Capablo, J.L.; Alfonso, P.; Garcia-Rodriguez, B.; Latre, P.; Irun, P.; de Cabezon, A.S.; Pocovi, M. Neurological manifestations in patients with Gaucher disease and their relatives, it is just a coincidence? *J. Inherit. Metab. Dis.* **2011**, *34*, 781–787. [CrossRef] [PubMed]
43. Setó-Salvia, N.; Pagonabarraga, J.; Houlden, H.; Pascual-Sedano, B.; Dols-Icardo, O.; Tucci, A.; Paisán-Ruiz, C.; Campolongo, A.; Antón-Aguirre, S.; Martín, I.; et al. Glucocerebrosidase mutations confer a greater risk of dementia during Parkinson's disease course. *Mov. Disord.* **2012**, *27*, 393–399. [CrossRef] [PubMed]
44. Sun, Y.; Grabowski, G.A. Impaired autophagosomes and lysosomes in neuronopathic Gaucher disease. *Autophagy* **2010**, *6*, 648–649. [CrossRef] [PubMed]
45. Wang, Y.; Zhang, H.W.; Ye, J.; Qiu, W.J.; Han, L.S.; Gu, X.F. Comparison and clinical application of two methods for determination of plasma chitotriosidase activity. *Zhonghua Er Ke Za Zhi* **2012**, *50*, 834–838. (In Chinese)
46. Choi, J.M.; Kim, W.C.; Lyoo, C.H.; Kang, S.Y.; Lee, P.H.; Baik, J.S.; Koh, S.B.; Ma, H.I.; Sohn, Y.H.; Lee, M.S.; et al. Association of mutations in the glucocerebrosidase gene with Parkinson disease in a Korean population. *Neurosci. Lett.* **2012**, *514*, 12–15. [CrossRef]
47. Biegstraaten, M.; Wesnes, K.A.; Luzy, C.; Petakov, M.; Mrsic, M.; Niederau, C.; Giraldo, P.; Hughes, D.; Mehta, A.; Mengel, K.E.; et al. The cognitive profile of type 1 Gaucher disease patients. *J. Inherit. Metab. Dis.* **2012**, *35*, 1093–1099. [CrossRef] [PubMed]
48. Schapira, A.H. Glucocerebrosidase and Parkinson disease: Recent advances. *Mol. Cell Neurosci.* **2015**, *66*, 37–42. [CrossRef] [PubMed]
49. Barrett, M.J.; Hagenah, J.; Dhawan, V.; Peng, S.; Stanley, K.; Raymond, D.; Deik, A.; Gross, S.J.; Schreiber-Agus, N.; Mirelman, A.; et al. LRRK2 Ashkenazi Jewish Consortium. Transcranial sonography and functional imaging in glucocerebrosidase mutation Parkinson disease. *Parkinsonism Relat. Disord.* **2013**, *19*, 186–191. [CrossRef] [PubMed]
50. Saunders-Pullman, R.; Hagenah, J.; Dhawan, V.; Stanley, K.; Pastores, G.; Sathe, S.; Tagliati, M.; Condefer, K.; Palmese, C.; Brüggemann, N.; et al. Gaucher disease ascertained through a Parkinson's center: Imaging and clinical characterization. *Mov. Disord.* **2010**, *25*, 1364–1372. [CrossRef]
51. Goker-Alpan, O.; Masdeu, J.C.; Kohn, P.D.; Ianni, A.; Lopez, G.; Groden, C.; Chapman, M.C.; Cropp, B.; Eisenberg, D.P.; Maniwang, E.D.; et al. The neurobiology of glucocerebrosidase-associated parkinsonism: A positron emission tomography study of dopamine synthesis and regional cerebral blood flow. *Brain* **2012**, *135*, 2440–2448. [CrossRef]
52. Agosta, F.; Sarasso, E.; Filippi, M. Functional MRI in Atypical Parkinsonisms. *Int. Rev. Neurobiol.* **2018**, *142*, 149–173. [CrossRef] [PubMed]
53. Kraoua, I.; Stirnemann, J.; Ribeiro, M.J.; Rouaud, T.; Verin, M.; Annic, A.; Rose, C.; Defebvre, L.; Réménieras, L.; Schüpbach, M.; et al. Parkinsonism in Gaucher's disease type 1: Ten new cases and a review of the literature. *Mov. Disord.* **2009**, *24*, 1524–1530. [CrossRef] [PubMed]
54. Parnetti, L.; Paciotti, S.; Eusebi, P.; Dardis, A.; Zampieri, S.; Chiasserini, D.; Tasegian, A.; Tambasco, N.; Bembi, B.; Calabresi, P.; et al. Cerebrospinal fluid β-glucocerebrosidase activity is reduced in parkinson's disease patients. *Mov. Disord.* **2017**, *32*, 1423–1431. [CrossRef] [PubMed]
55. Parnetti, L.; Chiasserini, D.; Persichetti, E.; Eusebi, P.; Varghese, S.; Qureshi, M.M.; Dardis, A.; Deganuto, M.; De Carlo, C.; Castrioto, A.; et al. Cerebrospinal fluid lysosomal enzymes and alpha-synuclein in Parkinson's disease. *Mov. Disord.* **2014**, *29*, 1019–1027. [CrossRef] [PubMed]
56. Alcalay, R.N.; Levy, O.A.; Waters, C.C.; Fahn, S.; Ford, B.; Kuo, S.-H.; Mazzoni, P.; Pauciulo, M.W.; Nichols, W.C.; Gan-Or, Z.; et al. Glucocerebrosidase activity in Parkinson's disease with and without GBA mutations. *Brain* **2015**, *138*, 2648–2658. [CrossRef]
57. Gatto, E.M.; Etcheverry, J.L.; Sanguinetti, A.; Cesarini, M.; Fernandez Escobar, N.; Drelichman, G. Prodromal Clinical Markers of Parkinson disease in Gaucher Disease Individuals. *Eur. Neurol.* **2016**, *76*, 19–21. [CrossRef] [PubMed]

58. Litvan, I.; Goldman, J.G.; Tröster, A.I.; Schmand, B.A.; Weintraub, D.; Petersen, R.C.; Mollenhauer, B.; Adler, C.H.; Marder, K.; Williams-Gray, C.H.; et al. Diagnostic criteria for mild cognitive impairment in Parkinson's disease: Movement Disorder Society Task Force guidelines. *Mov. Disord.* **2012**, *27*, 349–356. [CrossRef]
59. Liu, G.; Locascio, J.J.; Corvol, J.C.; Boot, B.; Liao, Z.; Page, K.; Franco, D.; Burke, K.; Jansen, I.E.; Trisini-Lipsanopoulos, A.; et al. Prediction of cognition in Parkinson's disease with a clinical-genetic score: A longitudinal analysis of nine cohorts. *Lancet Neurol.* **2017**, *16*, 620–629. [CrossRef]
60. Mata, I.F.; Leverenz, J.B.; Weintraub, D.; Trojanowski, J.Q.; Chen-Plotkin, A.; Van Deerlin, V.M.; Ritz, B.; Rausch, R.; Factor, S.A.; Wood-Siverio, C.; et al. GBA Variants are associated with a distinct pattern of cognitive deficits in Parkinson's disease. *Mov. Disord.* **2016**, *31*, 95–102. [CrossRef]
61. Bregman, N.; Thaler, A.; Mirelman, A.; Helmich, R.C.; Gurevich, T.; Orr-Urtreger, A.; Marder, K.; Bressman, S.; Bloem, B.R.; Giladi, N. LRRK2 Ashkenazi Jewish consortium. A cognitive fMRI study in non-manifesting LRRK2 and GBA carriers. *Brain Struct. Funct.* **2017**, *222*, 1207–1218. [CrossRef]
62. Chahine, L.M.; Urbe, L.; Caspell-Garcia, C.; Aarsland, D.; Alcalay, R.; Barone, P.; Burn, D.; Espay, A.J.; Hamilton, J.L.; Hawkins, K.A.; et al. Parkinson's Progression Markers Initiative. Cognition among individuals along a spectrum of increased risk for Parkinson's disease. *PLoS ONE* **2018**, *20*, e0201964. [CrossRef]
63. Taguchi, Y.V.; Liu, J.; Ruan, J.; Pacheco, J.; Zhang, X.; Abbasi, J.; Keutzer, J.; Mistry, P.K.; Chandra, S.S. Glucosylsphingosine Promotes α-Synuclein Pathology in MutantGBA-Associated Parkinson's Disease. *J. Neurosci.* **2017**, *37*, 9617–9631. [CrossRef] [PubMed]
64. Chun, Y.; Kim, J. Autophagy: An Essential Degradation Program for Cellular Homeostasis and Life. *Cells* **2018**, *7*, 278. [CrossRef] [PubMed]
65. Levine, B.; Kroemer, G. Biological Functions of Autophagy Genes: A Disease Perspective. *Cell* **2019**, *176*, 11–42. [CrossRef] [PubMed]
66. Bengoa-Vergniory, N.; Roberts, R.F.; Wade-Martins, R.; Alegre-Abarrategui, J. Alpha-synuclein oligomers: A new hope. *Acta Neuropathol.* **2017**, *134*, 819–838. [CrossRef] [PubMed]
67. Mor, D.E.; Daniels, M.J.; Ischiropoulos, H. The usual suspects, dopamine and alpha-synuclein, conspire to cause neurodegeneration. *Mov. Disord.* **2019**. [CrossRef]
68. Blandini, F.; Cilia, R.; Cerri, S.; Pezzoli, G.; Schapira, A.H.V.; Mullin, S.; Lanciego, J.L. Glucocerebrosidase mutations and synucleinopathies: Toward a model of precision medicine. *Mov. Disord.* **2018**. [CrossRef]
69. Ruskey, J.A.; Greenbaum, L.; Roncière, L.; Alam, A.; Spiegelman, D.; Liong, C.; Levy, O.A.; Waters, C.; Fahn, S.; Marder, K.S.; et al. Increased yield of full GBA sequencing in Ashkenazi Jews with Parkinson's disease. *Eur. J. Med. Genet.* **2018**, S1769–S7212. [CrossRef]
70. Stirnemann, J.; Vigan, M.; Hamroun, D.; Heraoui, D.; Rossi-Semerano, L.; Berger, M.G.; Rose, C.; Camou, F.; de Roux-Serratrice, C.; Grosbois, B.; et al. The French Gaucher's disease registry: Clinical characteristics, complications and treatment of 562 patients. *Orphanet J. Rare Dis.* **2012**, *7*, 77. [CrossRef]
71. Liu, G.; Boot, B.; Locascio, J.J.; Jansen, I.E.; Winder-Rhodes, S.; Eberly, S.; Elbaz, A.; Brice, A.; Ravina, B.; van Hilten, J.J.; et al. Specifically neuropathic Gaucher's mutations accelerate cognitive decline in Parkinson's. *Ann. Neurol.* **2016**, *80*, 674–685. [CrossRef]
72. Zhang, Y.; Shu, L.; Sun, Q.; Zhou, X.; Pan, H.; Guo, J.; Tang, B. Integrated Genetic Analysis of Racial Differences of Common GBA Variants in Parkinson's Disease: A Meta-Analysis. *Front. Mol. Neurosci.* **2018**, *11*, 43. [CrossRef] [PubMed]
73. Huang, Y.; Deng, L.; Zhong, Y.; Yi, M. The Association between E326K of GBA and the Risk of Parkinson's Disease. *Parkinsons Dis.* **2018**, *2018*, 1048084. [CrossRef] [PubMed]
74. Zhang, Y.; Sun, Q.Y.; Zhao, Y.W.; Shu, L.; Guo, J.F.; Xu, Q.; Yan, X.X.; Tang, B.S. Effect of GBA Mutations on Phenotype of Parkinson's Disease: A Study on Chinese Population and a Meta-Analysis. *Parkinsons Dis.* **2015**, *2015*, 916971. [CrossRef] [PubMed]
75. Bustamante, H.A.; González, A.E.; Cerda-Troncoso, C.; Shaughnessy, R.; Otth, C.; Soza, A.; Burgos, P.V. Interplay Between the Autophagy-Lysosomal Pathway and the Ubiquitin-Proteasome System: A Target for Therapeutic Development in Alzheimer's Disease. *Front. Cell. Neurosci.* **2018**, *12*, 126. [CrossRef] [PubMed]
76. Pitcairn, C.; Wani, W.Y.; Mazzolli, J. Dysregulation of the autophagic-lysosomal pathway in Gaucher Disease and Parkinson's Disease. *Neurobiol. Dis.* **2018**, *122*, 72–82. [CrossRef] [PubMed]

77. Braak, H.; Del Tredici, K.; Rüb, U.; de Vos, R.A.; Jansen Steur, E.N.; Braak, E. Staging of brain pathology related to sporadic Parkinson's disease. *Neurobiol. Aging* **2003**, *24*, 197–211. [CrossRef]
78. Gegg, M.E.; Schapira, A.H.V. The role of glucocerebrosidase in Parkinson disease pathogenesis. *FEBS J.* **2018**, *285*, 3591–3603. [CrossRef] [PubMed]
79. Zunke, F.; Andresen, L.; Wesseler, S.; Groth, J.; Arnold, P.; Rothaug, M.; Mazzulli, J.R.; Krainc, D.; Blanz, J.; Saftig, P.; et al. Characterization of the complex formed by β-glucocerebrosidase and the lysosomal integral membrane protein type-2. *Proc. Natl. Acad. Sci. USA* **2016**, *113*, 3791–3796. [CrossRef] [PubMed]
80. Mazzulli, J.R.; Xu, Y.H.; Sun, Y.; Knight, A.L.; McLean, P.J.; Caldwell, G.A.; Sidransky, E.; Grabowski, G.A.; Krainc, D. Gaucher disease glucocerebrosidase and α-synuclein form a bidirectional pathogenic loop in synucleinopathies. *Cell* **2011**, *146*, 37–52. [CrossRef] [PubMed]
81. Magalhaes, J.; Gegg, M.E.; Migdalska-Richards, A.; Doherty, M.K.; Whitfield, P.D.; Schapira, A.H. Autophagic lysosome reformation dysfunction in glucocerebrosidase deficient cells: Relevance to Parkinson disease. *Hum. Mol. Genet.* **2016**, *25*, 3432–3445. [CrossRef] [PubMed]
82. Thomas, R.E.; Vincow, E.S.; Merrihew, G.E.; MacCoss, M.J.; Davis, M.Y.; Pallanck, L.J. Glucocerebrosidase deficiency promotes protein aggregation through dysregulation of extracellular vesicles. *PLoS Genet.* **2018**, *14*, e1007694. [CrossRef] [PubMed]
83. Berthet, A.; Margolis, E.B.; Zhang, J.; Hsieh, I.; Zhang, J.; Hnasko, T.S.; Ahmad, J.; Edwards, R.H.; Sesaki, H.; Huang, E.J.; et al. Loss of mitochondrial fission depletes axonal mitochondria in midbrain dopamine neurons. *J. Neurosci.* **2014**, *34*, 14304–14317. [CrossRef] [PubMed]
84. Poole, A.C.; Thomas, R.E.; Andrews, L.A.; McBride, H.M.; Whitworth, A.J.; Pallanck, L.J. The PINK1/Parkin pathway regulates mitochondrial morphology. *Proc. Natl. Acad. Sci. USA* **2008**, *105*, 1638–1643. [CrossRef] [PubMed]
85. Wang, X.; Petrie, T.G.; Liu, Y.; Liu, J.; Fujioka, H.; Zhu, X. Parkinson's disease-associated DJ-1 mutations impair mitochondrial dynamics and cause mitochondrial dysfunction. *J. Neurochem.* **2012**, *121*, 830–839. [CrossRef] [PubMed]
86. Wang, X.; Yan, M.H.; Fujioka, H.; Liu, J.; Wilson-Delfosse, A.; Chen, S.G.; Perry, G.; Casadesus, G.; Zhu, X. LRRK2 regulates mitochondrial dynamics and function through direct interaction with DLP1. *Hum. Mol. Genet.* **2012**, *21*, 1931–1944. [CrossRef] [PubMed]
87. Kamp, F.; Exner, N.; Lutz, A.K.; Wender, N.; Hegermann, J.; Brunner, B.; Nuscher, B.; Bartels, T.; Giese, A.; Beyer, K.; et al. Inhibition of mitochondrial fusion by α-synuclein is rescued by PINK1, Parkin and DJ-1. *EMBO J.* **2010**, *29*, 3571–3589. [CrossRef]
88. Yun, S.P.; Kim, D.; Kim, S.; Kim, S.; Karuppagounder, S.S.; Kwon, S.H.; Lee, S.; Kam, T.I.; Lee, S.; Ham, S.; et al. α-Synuclein accumulation and GBA deficiency due to L444P GBA mutation contributes to MPTP-induced parkinsonism. *Mol. Neurodegener.* **2018**, *13*. [CrossRef]
89. Bendikov-Bar, I.; Rapaport, D.; Larisch, S.; Horowitz, M. Parkin-mediated ubiquitination of mutant glucocerebrosidase leads to competition with its substrates PARIS and ARTS. *Orphanet J. Rare Dis.* **2014**, *9*, 86. [CrossRef]
90. Li, H.; Ham, A.; Ma, T.C.; Kuo, S.H.; Kanter, E.; Kim, D.; Ko, H.S.; Quan, Y.; Sardi, S.P.; Li, A.; et al. Mitochondrial dysfunction and mitophagy defect triggered by heterozygous GBA mutations. *Autophagy* **2019**, *15*, 113–130. [CrossRef]
91. Stirnemann, J.; Belmatoug, N.; Camou, F.; Serratrice, C.; Froissart, R.; Caillaud, C.; Levade, T.; Astudillo, L.; Serratrice, J.; Brassier, A.; et al. A Review of Gaucher Disease Pathophysiology, Clinical Presentation and Treatments. *Int. J. Mol. Sci.* **2017**, *18*, 441. [CrossRef]
92. Extracted from Clinical Trials. Available online: clinicaltrials.gov/ct2/show/NCT02906020 (accessed on 11 December 2018).
93. Sardi, S.P.; Viel, C.; Clarke, J.; Treleaven, C.M.; Richards, A.M.; Park, H.; Olszewski, M.A.; Dodge, J.C.; Marshall, J.; Makino, E.; et al. GCS inhibitor treats synucleinopathy models. *Proc. Natl. Acad. Sci. USA* **2017**, *114*, 2699–2704. [CrossRef] [PubMed]
94. McNeill, A.; Magalhaes, J.; Shen, C.; Chau, K.Y.; Hughes, D.; Mehta, A.; Foltynie, T.; Cooper, J.M.; Abramov, A.Y.; Gegg, M.; et al. Ambroxol improves lysosomal biochemistry in glucocerebrosidase mutation-linked Parkinson disease cells. *Brain* **2014**, *137*, 1481–1495. [CrossRef] [PubMed]

95. Aflaki, E.; Borger, D.K.; Moaven, N.; Stubblefield, B.K.; Rogers, S.A.; Patnaik, S.; Schoenen, F.J.; Westbroek, W.; Zheng, W.; Sullivan, P.; et al. A New Glucocerebrosidase Chaperone Reduces α-Synuclein and Glycolipid Levels in iPSC-Derived Dopaminergic Neurons from Patients with Gaucher Disease and Parkinsonism. *J. Neurosci.* **2016**, *36*, 7441–7452. [CrossRef] [PubMed]
96. Mistry, P.K.; Lopez, G.; Schiffmann, R.; Barton, N.W.; Weinreb, N.J.; Sidransky, E. 27 Progress and ongoing challenges. *Mol. Genet. Metab.* **2016**, *120*, 8–21. [CrossRef] [PubMed]
97. Zunke, F.; Moise, A.C.; Belur, N.R.; Gelyana, E.; Stojkovska, I.; Dzaferbegovic, H.; Toker, N.J.; Jeon, S.; Fredriksen, K.; Mazzulli, J.R. Reversible Conformational Conversion of α-Synuclein into Toxic Assemblies by Glucosylceramide. *Neuron* **2018**, *97*, 92–107. [CrossRef] [PubMed]
98. Kim, M.J.; Jeon, S.; Burbulla, L.F.; Krainc, D. Acid ceramidase inhibition ameliorates α-synuclein accumulation upon loss of GBA1 function. *Hum. Mol. Genet.* **2018**, *27*, 1972–1988. [CrossRef] [PubMed]
99. Espay, A.J.; Brundin, P.; Lang, A.E. Precision medicine for disease modification in Parkinson disease. *Nat. Rev. Neurol.* **2017**, *13*, 119–126. [CrossRef] [PubMed]

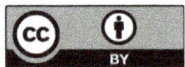 © 2019 by the authors. Licensee MDPI, Basel, Switzerland. This article is an open access article distributed under the terms and conditions of the Creative Commons Attribution (CC BY) license (http://creativecommons.org/licenses/by/4.0/).

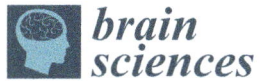

Review

The Genetic Diagnosis of Neurodegenerative Diseases and Therapeutic Perspectives

Julio-César García [1,2,*] and Rosa-Helena Bustos [1]

1. Evidence-Based Therapeutics Group, Department of Clinical Pharmacology, Universidad de La Sabana, Chía 140013, Colombia; rosa.bustos@unisabana.edu.co
2. Department of Clinical Pharmacology, Clínica Universidad de La Sabana, Chía 140013, Colombia
* Correspondence: julio.garcia@unisabana.edu.co; Tel.: +57-1861-5555

Received: 11 October 2018; Accepted: 7 December 2018; Published: 13 December 2018

Abstract: Genetics has led to a new focus regarding approaches to the most prevalent diseases today. Ascertaining the molecular secrets of neurodegenerative diseases will lead to developing drugs that will change natural history, thereby affecting the quality of life and mortality of patients. The sequencing of candidate genes in patients suffering neurodegenerative pathologies is faster, more accurate, and has a lower cost, thereby enabling algorithms to be proposed regarding the risk of neurodegeneration onset in healthy persons including the year of onset and neurodegeneration severity. Next generation sequencing has resulted in an explosion of articles regarding the diagnosis of neurodegenerative diseases involving exome sequencing or sequencing a whole gene for correlating phenotypical expression with genetic mutations in proteins having key functions. Many of them occur in neuronal glia, which can trigger a proinflammatory effect leading to defective proteins causing sporadic or familial mutations. This article reviews the genetic diagnosis techniques and the importance of bioinformatics in interpreting results from neurodegenerative diseases. Risk scores must be established in the near future regarding diseases with a high incidence in healthy people for defining prevention strategies or an early start for giving drugs in the absence of symptoms.

Keywords: genetic biomarker; Parkinson's disease (PD); Alzheimer's disease (AD); next generation sequencing (NGS); diagnosis; neurodegenerative disease; amyotrophic lateral sclerosis (ALS)

---

1. Introduction

Advances have been made regarding chronic disease therapy due to an understanding of altered molecular mechanisms in cells from different bodily organs. One of the most fascinating advances during the last decade has occurred in the field of genetics concerning new sequencing techniques; this concerns identifying genotypic aberrations leading to the determination dysfunctional phenotypic expressions using large bioinformatic databases. Sequencing a genome or exome for clinical applications has now entered medical practice. Several thousand tests have already been ordered for patients to establish a diagnosis regarding rare diseases that are clinically unrecognizable, or baffling, but have a suspected genetic origin.

Neurological diseases are disorders of the brain, spinal cord, and the nerves. There are more than 600 neurological diseases [1], the major types being genetic (such as Huntington's disease); developmental disorders (i.e., cerebral palsy and spina bifida); degenerative diseases (i.e., Alzheimer's disease (AD) and Parkinson's disease (PD)); cerebrovascular diseases (i.e., stroke); physical injuries to the brain, spinal cord, or nerves; seizure disorders (i.e., epilepsy); brain tumors (i.e., glioma); infection (i.e., meningitis); mental disorders such as affective and personality disorders (e.g., bipolar disorder and schizophrenia); sleep disorders (i.e., insomnia); and addictive disorders (i.e., alcoholism) [2].

The neuroinflammatory reaction caused by neurons and non-neuronal cells in neurodegenerative diseases (NDs) is persistent due to many triggering factors leading to the mutation of genes altering proteins implicated in the development of neurodegeneration such as the beta amyloid protein in AD, the alpha-synuclein protein in PD, and the superoxide dismutase (SOD)-1 mutation in amyotrophic lateral sclerosis (ALS), as discussed later on [3]. The selective expression in astrocytes and the microglia per se does not result in motor neurodegeneration [4,5], thereby implying a fundamental role for surrounding cells during neuron activation. Other studies have focused on the proinflammatory factor associated with microglial neurotoxicity by deleting factors such as TNF-alpha or interleukin beta as having a small effect on survival [6,7]. The biological processes promoting these reactions in the glia are complex and have harmful effects on the motor neurons. Therapeutical interventions directed against target cells are being explored. A better understanding of the biological and genetic processes implicated in neuroinflammation will help in defining their importance in ND physiopathology for identifying potential therapeutic interventions for detaining or differing reactions regarding neurodegeneration [8].

The field of neurology is not the exception in the explosion of articles/material proclaiming the usefulness of genetics in identifying genetic risk factors and regarding diagnosis specificity. NDs have been the target for intensive research in the field of genetics due to their great impact on morbimortality of adult patients. This article has thus been aimed at reviewing recent advances in the genetic diagnosis of the following ND: AD, PD, and ALS.

2. Obtaining Genetic Information

2.1. Sanger Sequencing

In 1977, Sanger et al. established the most commonly used method, until recently, for sequencing a determined fragment of deoxyribonucleic acid (DNA) [9]. It enabled around 500 base pairs to be sequenced with a 99% specificity; however, the technique is time-consuming for large sequences, such as in identifying NDs; therefore, new sequencing techniques have emerged. Sanger is the technique of choice for confirming point mutations found by other methods that could be related to the onset/appearance of a ND [10]. Figure 1 describes the procedure used for Sanger sequencing [11].

2.2. Next Generation Sequencing (NGS)

NGS incorporates technologies that produce millions of short DNA sequences at low cost and in a short time, read mostly in the 25 to 700 bp length range for a gene suspected of producing a disease [12]. It represents an efficient sequencing technique for multiple, short sequences in parallel so that multiple genes can be sequenced or even the complete human genome. Its main advantages lie in its rapid sequencing, low cost, and parallel sequencing of multiple genes [13–15]; its disadvantage lies in the exactitude of the results ranging from 93% to 99%, meaning that it is often thereby necessary to confirm such results by the Sanger technique. However, it is currently the most used technique due to its differential advantages. Whole genome sequencing (WGS) has been used for diagnosing NDs or just the encoding region or exome (i.e., whole exome sequencing (WES)) [16,17]. The large amount of data obtained by using these techniques has affected the development of informatics departments, leading to a change in the approach to molecular diagnosis, inverting the pyramid between technology and interpretation. The techniques most commonly used in diagnosing NDs will be reviewed later on.

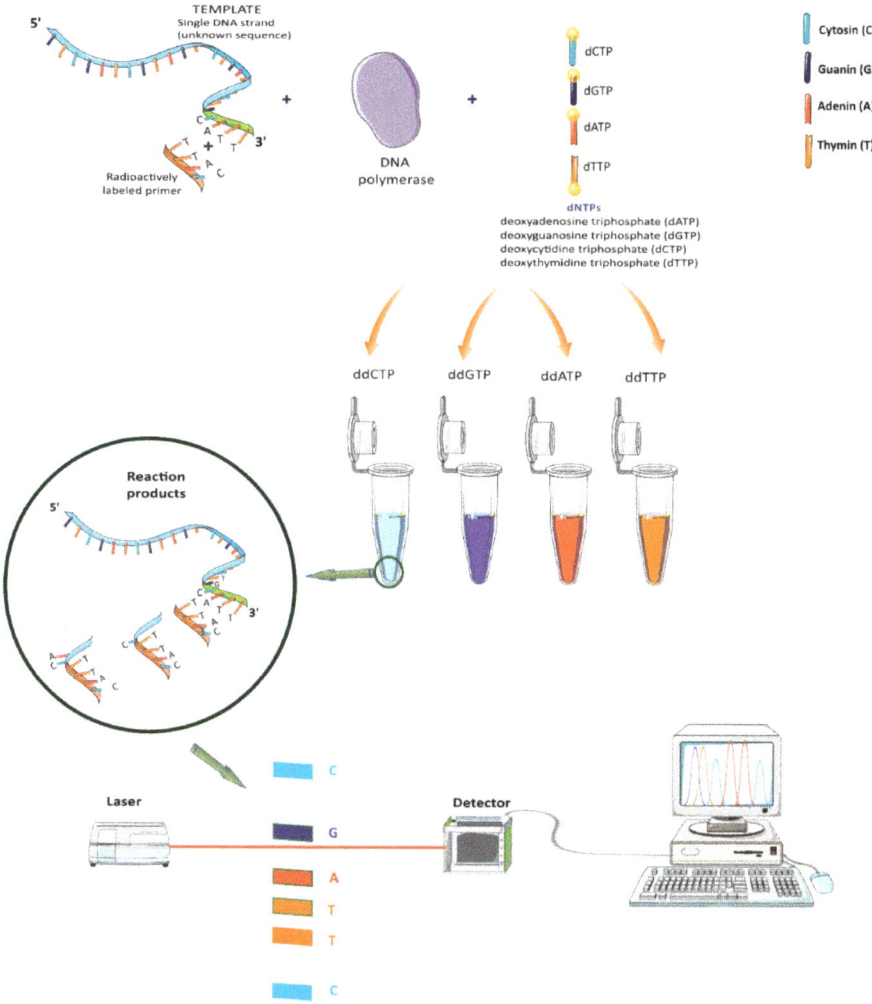

Figure 1. Sanger sequencing [11].

A person's DNA consists of more than 3000 million nucleotides in the genome, whilst the exome (the part of the genome which we "understand" is little more than 1% of the genome. Enriching the exome and sequencing, instead of the whole genome, continues to be the method of choice, essentially because it is cheaper [18]. However, several companies are rapidly moving toward sequencing the genome to provide greater coverage; this will facilitate processing more samples and avoiding expensive PCR artifacts.

The exome is the part of the genome which we think we understand including all the encoding regions (i.e., about 200,000 exons from 21,000 genes). An exome is little more than 1% of the genome; up to 85% of all mutations causing disease in Mendelian disorders are found within the encoding exons, thereby still being the most requested method [19]. WES is indicated when heterogeneous disorders are suspected (i.e., similar phenotypes in many genes) such as intellectual disability/developmental delay, epilepsy, muscular dystrophy, ataxia, neuropathy, deafness, or retinitis pigmentosa [20]. Regarding unclear phenotypes, the technique is also useful when a doctor may not recognize a patient's possible diagnosis (i.e., atypical clinical presentations). It is highly effective in identifying causal variants having short response times, thereby being economic, is impartial due to being able to evaluate thousands of genes simultaneously and the fact that dual diagnosis is possible [16,17].

DNA must be isolated and fragmented to enable sequencing the exome; the resulting DNA fragments are a mixture of introns and exons. The following step consists of separating the exons from the rest of the genome and sequencing them; the exome must be amplified, and during amplification, fragmented DNA becomes exposed to the surface containing the whole exome sequence. Then, the complementary regions (just exons) bind (making hybrids). The remaining DNA (introns) becomes eliminated in the process. Finally, the exons are sequenced and compared to a reference sequence; thousands of variants appear (around 60,000 per sample) from such a comparison. All the variants are filtered until the variants causing a particular disease are detected. Just exon variants can be selected from the 60,000 variants, thereby reducing the number of variants to be considered to 13,000. This process is repeated until just a few variants are obtained (about 10). It is then possible to observe which variants are shared with other members of a (target) family [14,15].

The disadvantages of WES can be divided into two groups: enrichment mechanisms and coverage difficulties. Regarding enrichment mechanisms, this is the most relevant inconvenience, especially because when "enriching" the exome by hybridization or amplification, not only are artifacts introduced into the sequencing and amplify the DNA by PCR, but elements also become introduced as not all of the regions can be amplified in the same pattern. Regarding coverage, difficulties arise due to enrichment measures and amplification addressing regions with weak coverage or regions lacking coverage, and various mutations not being found in the exome (e.g., a regulatory element) and not being able to be detected [15,17].

WGS will surely replace WES because of its reduced cost; from a methodological point of view, it is better to have fewer extras, have homogeneous coverage, and a better analysis strategy. Knowledge has been gained every day when evaluating elements related to parts of the genome which are unrelated to the exon. Other cases where using WES would be indicated would be an unclear phenotype, atypical clinical presentations, challenging cases regarding their interpretation, and evaluating results. Other cases would involve a negative result where the cost can be assumed and when a genetic diagnosis is required which involves cutting-edge technology [13,14,16,17]. Table 1 summarizes the differences between WES and WGS.

Table 1. Differences between whole-exome sequencing (WES) and WGS.

WES	WGS
Only done in encoding regions (exons)	Complete sequence: exons and introns
Cheap and fast	Currently expensive
Incomplete analysis of the target region	Technology-related challenges: an enormous amount of data is produced
Inclined towards known biology (medically-relevant genes)	Increased precision providing information about position and orientation

The Human Phenotype Ontology (HPO) project provides standardized terminology (more than 10,000 terms) regarding the phenotypical abnormalities found in human genetic syndromes. Phenotypical characteristics are formally represented as terms on a directed acyclic graph. Multiple paternity allows the representation of different aspects regarding phenotypical abnormalities [21]. The HPO's >10,000 integral, structured, and well-defined terms describe human phenotypical aberrations. It provides annotations concerning almost 7300 human hereditary syndromes, producing computable representations of the diseases, genes from associated diseases, signs, symptoms, paraclinical abnormalities, and other phenotypical anomalous characterizing distinct diseases including ND [22–24]. The authors index different algorithms from the HPO, constructed according to each investigation. The HPO data provide a powerful tool/resource for translational research, providing the means for capturing, storing, and exchanging phenotypical information about pathologies and has been used for integrating phenotypical information regarding computational analysis [21,22,25–27]. Research results using NGS (specifically WES and WGS), using clinical analysis for substantially improving candidate gene ranking, have enabled clinical evaluation based on bioinformatics analysis results to become integrated into the flow, thereby transforming phenotypical expression in candidate genes [21,28,29].

The strategy of filtering possible variants is designed to highlight rare or de novo mutations as well as high penetrance mutations modifying proteins. The filtering strategy substantially reduces the list of candidate variants found in expression concerning the confirmation of their functionality in an individual.

3. The Genetics of Neurodegenerative Diseases

Studies by Van Deerlin et al. discussed the importance of putting advances in genetic knowledge regarding NDs into practice, highlighting the correct use of nomenclature, changes in the approach to identified variants, ethical aspects arising from managing the information, the resources available for accessing information, and the genetic counselling that patients and their families-care-givers should receive regarding the diagnosis of a disease having a defined inheritance pattern [30].

Identifying mutations in ND-related genes is important regarding different areas of knowledge such as basic research, clinical research, clinical characteristics, and identifying biomarkers and images. The scope of this article focused on identifying the mutations related to each disease.

3.1. Alzheimer's Disease (AD)

The main cause of dementia affects around 35 million patients around the world [31]; it is produced by the accumulation of various forms of amyloid proteins and neurofibrillary degeneration [32,33]. Evidence has been presented stating that 58% to 79% of dementias have a genetic component [34]. Inherited family traits have been reported since 1930; they can be explained by an autosomal dominant model, i.e., 50% risk in the following generation of having a mutation in the amyloid precursor protein (APP), presenilin 1 (PSEN1), and/or presenilin 2 (PSEN2) genes [33].

The APP gene's official name is the amyloid beta 4 (A4) precursor protein; APP is mainly found in the CNS. Kang et al. cloned the gene from chromosome 21 [35,36]. Ryman et al. identified the factors influencing onset age, onset of symptoms, and the course of autosomal dominant AD including the Dominantly Inherited Alzheimer Network's (DIAN) databases, involving two large families from Colombia (PSEN 1, E280A) and Germany (PSEN 2, Nl41l). A total of 1307 patients were included who have had a diagnosis of AD; 174 familial mutations were found that correlated with the disease's onset age [36,37].

Most variants with an identified risk in more than 20 genes, determined by genome-wide association studies (GWAS), have not been recognized as affecting protein structure or function, only conferring 10% to 20% of risk of disease [38]. Other variants in genes have been previously identified that are not related to AD such as TREM2, UNC 5C, and/or AKAP9; these have a similar effect on the risk of AD regarding allele APOE E4 [39–42].

APOE, a component of senile plaques [43], has been seen to influence neuritic plaque formation in models of transgenic mice suffering AD and is also considered to contribute toward AB clearance and its deposition in the brain [44]. Other in vitro and in vivo studies have suggested that APOE participates in synaptogenesis, cognition, neurotoxicity, Tau hyperphosphorylation, neuroinflammation, and cerebral metabolism. APOE e4 is a genetic risk factor that is neither necessary nor sufficient for AD development [45].

Identifying single-nucleotide polymorphisms (SNP) in the human genome and the development of SNP genotyping technologies have led to the genetic understanding of commonly occurring complex diseases [46,47]. More than 600 candidate genes have been studied regarding AD development; these are regularly updated at the AlzGene website [47,48]. These studies have led to genes such as the sortilin-related receptor (SORL1) [49] and calcium homeostasis modulator 1 (CALHM1) being identified [50], however, the main problems with these genes are the false positives, false negatives, and heterogeneity in phenotypes, genotypes and potential gene–gene and gene–environment interaction [48,51,52].

GWAS use large platforms consisting of different SNP markers; it is worth mentioning late onset AD association studies [53]. GWAS has identified the following candidate genes: the galanin-like peptide precursor (GALP) [54], phosphoenolpyruvate carboxykinase 1 (PCK1) [55], trafficking kinesin-binding protein 2 (TRAK2) [54], tyrosine kinase non-receptor 1 (TNK1) [54], the GRB-associated binding protein 2 (GAB2) [56], Golgi phosphoprotein 2 (GOLPH2) [57], lecithin retinol acyltransferase (LRAT) [58], and protocadherin 11X (PCDH11X) [59]. Other genes include TRPC4AP, CLU, PICALM, CR1, LMNA, THEMS, MAPT, and CH25H [54,55,60–62]. Studies have revealed the population attributable risk (PAR) and association (OR) between the gene presence and AD development via the relationship with APOE: TOMM40 (OR 2.73, PAR 20.6%) and APOC1 (OR 4.01, PAR 35.1%) [33,54,63].

The clinical implications of genetic discoveries have been mentioned in different studies [52,64,65] with greater interest being shown in APOE and SORL1, giving a 33% risk for males and 32% for females aged 75-years old, whilst this rose to 52% for males over 85 and 68% for females over 85-years old (Table 2). Only 2% of the Caucasian population have the APOE e4/e4 genotype; screening for APOE has not yet been recommended, but will soon be necessary with the new genetic markers.

Table 2. Dominant autosomal genes regarding AD [33].

Gene	Symbol	Inheritance	Location	Risk (%)
Amyloid precursor protein	APP	Autosomal dominant	21q21.3	38–69
Presenilin 1	PSEN1	Autosomal dominant	14q24.2	25–65
Presenilin 2	PSEN2	Autosomal dominant, reduced penetrance	1q42.13	41–88

3.2. Amyotrophic Lateral Sclerosis (ALS)

Amyotrophic lateral sclerosis (or Lou Gehrig's disease) is one of the main NDs of the motor neurons, leading to death within 3 to 5 years following the onset of symptoms. Its prevalence is 1 in 300 people and produces large-scale disability in patients suffering from it. Superoxide dismutase Cu/Zn or SOD1 was the first ALS-associated gene to be identified in 1993 [66]. Recent advances in genetic diagnosis have led to discovering other genetic markers using GWAS; familial inheritance occurs in 5% to 20%. Current knowledge states that more than 20 genes are correlated with the onset of ALS. The guidelines for the molecular diagnosis of neurogenetic disorders [67] refer to diseases having greater evidence from genetic exams including familial ALS, bulbar muscular atrophy, Charcot-Marie-Tooth neuropathy type 1A, myotonic dystrophy, and Duchenne muscular dystrophy.

Even though GWAS has broadened the panorama of genes in different diseases like ALS, other factors associated with the onset of NDs have been reported in studies on twins and families having established hereditary components. Further in-depth studies are needed into the genetics as well as into polygenetics and epigenetics to ensure personalized medicine by finding the factors triggering diseases [68–70].

Evidence regarding genetic traits in ALS has emerged from studies on twins, demonstrating the inheritance in the onset of sporadic ALS, ranging from 0.38 to 0.78 (heritability value) [71,72]. However, in addition to the above, two situations hamper the identification of genes in ALS; initially, the disease is late onset, thereby avoiding the characterization of lineages and prognosis is poor, thereby hampering follow-up and requiring multicenter studies for sample taking [73–75]. Al-Chalabi et al. provided a simple explanation for the relationship between genetics and the disease's pathology, stressing the presence of protein inclusions in the spinal motor neurons produced by mutated genes SOD1, TDP43, FUS, and/or OPTN [76].

In 2014, Keller et al. estimated important genetic factors by meta-analysis using GWES databases, and found a 21% probability of inheritance, identifying 17 regions of the genome having high significance for the disease [77]. Interestingly, they estimated a 35% inheritance in patients having a bulbar presentation, more than 40% inherited cases, and 20% sporadic cases for the hexanucleotide repeat expansion in C9ORF72 located on the short arm of chromosome 9. Other studies have shown consistent expansion (hundreds of times) in (GGGGCC), causing neuron loss in the anterior horn of the spinal cord causing cellular inclusions similar to TDP-43 [78].

The genes related to familial inheritance in ALS (in order of importance) are SOD1, encoding a copper/zinc superoxide dismutase [66,76] whose alteration produces cytotoxicity, mitochondrial dysfunction, oxidative stress, axonal aberrations, and is involved in endosome traffic [79–85]. TARDBP encodes the TDP-43 protein involved in RNA splicing [78]; its alteration produces neuron loss, gliosis, and Bunin body inclusions in the spinal column's anterior horn [86,87]. FUS encodes a sarcoma protein related to RNA processing whose cerebral and spinal mutation causes severe motor neuron loss in the spinal column [88,89]. UBQLN2 encodes a protein similar to ubiquitin [90], which is responsible for ubiquitin-mediated protein degradation, whose mutation is X-linked; males suffer from the disease more frequently than females who have a certain degree of protection [91,92]. TATA-Box Binding Protein Associated Factor 15 (TAF15) is linked to changes in the TATA-binding protein associated with factor 15 [93].

The unc-13 homolog A (UNC13A), elongator acetyltransferase complex subunit 3 (ELP3), homeostatic iron regulator (HFE), angiogenin (ANG), neurofilament heavy (NEFH), and EWS RNA binding protein 1 (EWSR1) genes have been reported to be associated with sporadic ALS [84,94–101], as have genes associated with familiar inheritance such as *TAF15* [101], *C9orf72* [102], *C21orf2*, myelin-associated oligodendrocyte basic protein (MOBP), and SCDF1 [103]. Recent WES exome sequencing has led to finding genes like TANK-binding kinase 1 (TBK1) [104].

Different studies have been carried out on chimeric mice, leading to the inclusion of the SOD1 gene: they have shown cell complex pathways and molecular injury at neuromuscular junctions and in the cell body of the motor neurons [105–110]. Animal model histology has revealed the destruction of neuromuscular junctions, whilst numerous inclusions, proximal axon inflammation, mitochondrial inflammation, vacuoles, and neurofilament accumulations appear in patients [108]. Inadequately folded proteins including the SOD1 gen protein, and phosphorylate fused neurofilaments in the sarcoma reflecting physiopathological changes in hereditary and non-hereditary disease [109,110].

The immune and glial cells of transgenic mice with the SOD1 gene affect motor neuron development, highlighting a multifactorial disease with different mechanisms leading to neuron injury, involving non-neuron cells such as astrocytes, oligodendrocytes, and microglia for its rapid progression [110]. Neuroinflammation is the cornerstone in the onset of differing NDs including AD, PD, multiple sclerosis, and HIV-associated encephalopathy due to intervention in the balance between neuroprotection and neurotoxicity [111–123].

Nicolas et al. identified a new gene associated with ALS such as the kinesin family member 5A (KIF5A) using GWAS. In this study, 20,876 cases of ALS were compared with 59,804 controls [124]. Mutations in the KIF5A for the appearance of hereditary spastic paraplegia and Charcot-Marie-Tooth Type 2 occur in the N-terminal domain, while for ALS they are located in the C-terminal portion causing defects in the cytoskeleton. This is one of the mechanisms associated with the appearance of ALS together with alterations in RNA processing and protein homeostasis. The relationship between the mechanism and the genes associated with ALS are presented in Table 3.

Table 3. Altered pathways in ALS.

Mechanism	Mutated Genes
Dynamics of the cytoskeleton	PFN1, TUBA4A, DCTN1, and KIF5A
RNA processing	C9orf72, TDP-43, FUS, and MATR3
Protein homeostasis	UBQLN2, VCP, OPTN, and VAPB

The UNC13A gene in the variant rs12608932 is associated with a lower survival in patients with ALS, according to the study by Diekstra et al. [125]. A total of 450 sporadic cases of ALS comparing survival with 524 controls were analyzed. The UNC13A gene encodes the unc-13 homolog A protein that is part of a family of presynaptic proteins in the brain. This protein is involved in the regulation of the release of neurotransmitters in the neuromuscular junction. Another possible gene for intervention as a possible therapeutic target is the rs2412208 gene of the calmodulin binding transcription activator 1 (CAMTA1) variant whose presence of the GG or GT genotype is associated with a reduction in survival over four months compared to the TT genotype [126]. The triggering receptor expressed on myeloid cells 2 (TREM2) variant (p.R47H, rs75932628) increases the risk of AD, but not of frontotemporal lobar degeneration (FTLD) in ALS and PD [127].

3.3. Parkinson's Disease (PD)

This is the second most common cause of progressive ND; it affects 30 to 190 patients in 100,000 inhabitants with an average age regarding symptom onset of 60-years old [128]. PD is characterized by motor symptoms such as bradykinesia, muscular rigidity, resting tremor, and (later on) aberrations when walking [129]. One of pathological characteristics of PD patients is the progressive loss pigmented dopaminergic neurons in the black substance (BS) and locus coeruleus, accompanied by alpha–synuclein-positive Lewy bodies in the remaining neurons [128]. Around 10% are familial cases, most being sporadic, having mutated genes that have been researched and associated with an increased risk of the disease's onset [128]. Animal models have been used for establishing two possible causes of PD: neurotoxicity and genetic models; the former includes models using pigs, showing BS neurodegeneration when using neurotoxins such as 6-hydroxydopamine (6-OHDA) or 1-methyl-4-phenyl-1,2,3,6-tetrahydropyridine (MPTP) [130–132]. Genetically modified pigs have been unsuccessfully used for identifying the genetic model; however Larsen et al. identified monogenic PD-associated porcine genes such as LRRK2 (PARK8) sharing a 90% identity with the human genes responsible for autosomal dominant forms of PD [133]. Other porcine genes are associated with autosomal recessive forms of PD, but do not fall within the scope of this review (i.e., FBX07, parkin, DJ-1) [134–136].

NGS technology has been used by several researchers for finding mutations in candidate genes in familial PD, both autosomal dominant and recessive ones having incomplete penetrance. Chartier-Harlin et al. [137] studied the exome of PD patients with an autosomal dominant pattern, finding mutations in EIF4G1. Zamprich et al. also studied the exome of an Austrian family with 16 affected members; they found a mutation in c.1858G>A (p.Asp620Asn) in VPS35 [138]. VPS35 is an interesting protein, since it is implicated in several Wnt signaling pathways in the biogenesis of lysosomes [139]. Given the nature of late onset PD, it is difficult to identify mutations that are related to the disease in different aged family members; however, once identified, they can provide important information for early diagnosis and treatment of this ND [140].

Genes identified with those to whom the risk of developing PD can be attributed, can be classified according to the disease's clinical presentations in cases of autosomal dominant and autosomal recessive PD [141]. The first autosomal dominant mutation alpha-synuclein (PARK 1 and 4) was discovered by Nussbaum et al. in 1997 through research on mutations in a large Italian-American family, finding a genetic lesion on the long arm of chromosome 4 [142]. Research has shown that this is the major component of Lewy bodies, a pathognomonic marker for all PD; it also produces severe familial forms and such proteins are present in all forms of PD, in cytoplasmic inclusions in multiple systemic atrophy, dementia with Lewy bodies, and other ND [141]. The main mutations found in alpha-synuclein are p.A53T, pA30P, and p.E46K, triplication of the SNCA locus. The most recent hypothesis deals with alpha-synuclein levels and disease severity and the disease's late onset possibly being due to small aberrations in the protein [143]. Another autosomal dominant mutation is the leucine-rich repeat kinase 2 (LRRK2 or PARK2), located in the pericentromer region of chromosome 12, having reported mutations p.R1441G, p.R1444C, p.Y1699C, p.I1122V, p.I2020T, p.L1114L, and pG2019S; it is responsible for around 2% of sporadic familial PD cases in different countries [141]. Recent dominant mutations are ATXN2, ATXN3, VPS35 (PARK17), GCH1, MAPT, DCTN1, and EIF4G1.

The autosomal recessive mutations are parkin (PARK2), DJ1 (PARK7), ATP13A2 (PARK9), FBXO7 (PARK15), and PLA2G6 (PARK14) (see Table 4) [141].

Table 4. Autosomal recessive mutations in PA [141].

Protein	Gene	Function	Location	Risk (%)
Parkin [144]	PARK2	Ubiquitin proteasome system	Cortex, hippocampus, basal ganglions and cerebellum	10% of early onset PD
Deglycase protein (DJ1) [145]	PARK7	Controlling cell cycle and oncogenesis	Basal nucleus neurons and astrocytes	Rare, early onset
PTEN 1-induced kinase [146]	PARK6	Neuroprotector function: mitochondria-dependent cell apoptosis	Distributed throughout different tissue	Rare, familial, appearing during the 40s and 50s

On the other hand, it is important to bear in mind that the genome that does not encode a protein can generate progression to a disease by affecting the normal expression of a gene. The therapeutic possibility of constructing oligonucleotic antisequencing of the exons is known. However, there are microRNAs, unions introns/exons, repetitive RNA, and a large number of non-conforming RNA [147]. Matsu et al. presented examples of diseases and the development of drugs or potential therapeutic targets of the different sequence varieties. In the case of large sequences of non-coding RNA (long noncoding RNA), they proposed a review of the FANTOMS, ENCODE, and NONCODE database as well as to determine the subcellular localization of the site of action of the sequence. Specifically, polycomb repressive complex-2 (PRC2) [148] has been investigated as a regulator of genetic expression that includes various proteins that modify chromatin and inactivation of the chromosome [149]. Even the non-coding genome is little understood but present in survival associated mitochondrial melanoma specific oncogenic non-coding RNA [150] (SAMMSON), Angelman's syndrome [151] (alteration of the UBE3A gene expression), and metastasis-associated lung adenocarcinoma transcript 1 (MALAT1) [152]. Regarding its presence in neurodegenerative diseases, Wang et al. [153] summarized the long noncoding RNA associated with AD are BACE1-AS, BC200, 17A, NAT-Rad18, 51A, and GDNFOS; while those described in PD are NaPINK1, AS Uchl1, HOTAIR, and MALAT1; and in ELA C9ORF72, FUS/TLS, and TDP43.

4. Conclusions and Perspectives

Genetic tests for diagnosis or detection are necessary for detecting a genetic alteration/aberration in an affected person or one at risk. Test capacity for/ability to detect a genetic alteration depends on many factors including gene location, the nature of the mutation, test sensitivity (false negatives), test specificity (false positives), and reproducibility (including between run, within run, and with different operators) [154]. There are guidelines for the interpretation of germline multiple variants by means of criteria to classify the variants as pathogenic, probable pathogenic, uncertain significance, likely benign, or benign. However, these guidelines have some limitations and there is subjectivity in its interpretation. Future research should continue to be carried out on bioinformatics and technology increase. The challenge for clinical laboratories is to ensure that these tests can be integrated into clinical care [154,155]. There are still many questions concerning the bioinformatic analysis of sequence data including what should be the threshold for naming variants, what (type of) writing should be used to register a mutation, and which method should be used for predicting the consequences of a particular variant. [156]. The European Federation of Neurological Societies (EFNS) guidelines for managing ALS include DNA analysis for SOD1, SMN, SBMA, TDP43, and FUS amongst the recommended studies for diagnosing the disease, SOD1 mutation carriers are one of the diagnostic criteria, the use of riluzole in patients having the SOD1 mutation, the need for genetic exams in cases of a familial history of ALS, and sporadic cases having the phenotypical characteristics of the D90A recessive mutation. Genetic diagnosis is not recommended in cases of sporadic ALS with a classical typical phenotype. SOD1, TARDBP, FUS, or ANG determination is recommendable in familial or sporadic cases having an uncertain diagnosis [157]. All patients should receive genetic counselling before any genetic analysis is made and patients must sign an informed consent form regarding the same.

Author Contributions: R.H.B. and J.C.G. prepared the original draft. R.H.B. and J.C.G. wrote, reviewed, and edited the manuscript.

Funding: This review article received no external funding.

Acknowledgments: We would like to thank the Universidad de La Sabana for supporting our work and Jason Garry for carefully translating and revising the manuscript.

Conflicts of Interest: The authors declare no conflict of interest.

References

1. University of Maryland Medical System. Neurological Diseases and Movement Rehabilitation. Available online: https://www.umms.org/health-services/rehabilitation/services/neuro/neurological-diseases-movement-rehabilitation (accessed on 29 November 2018).
2. Verkhratsky, A.; Butt, A. Neuroglia in Neurological Diseases. In *Glial Physiology and Pathophysiology*; Wiley-Blackwell: West Sussex, UK, 2013; pp. 453–504.
3. Hanisch, U.K.; Kettenmann, H. Microglia: Active sensor and versatile effector cells in the normal and pathologic brain. *Nat. Neurosci.* **2007**, *10*, 1387–1394. [CrossRef] [PubMed]
4. Beers, D.R.; Henkel, J.S.; Xiao, Q.; Zhao, W.; Wang, J.; Yen, A.A.; Siklos, L.; McKercher, S.R.; Appel, S.H. Wild-type microglia extend survival in PU.1 knockout mice with familial amyotrophic lateral sclerosis. *Proc. Natl. Acad. Sci. USA* **2006**, *103*, 16021–16026. [CrossRef] [PubMed]
5. Gong, Y.H.; Parsadanian, A.S.; Andreeva, A.; Snider, W.D.; Elliott, J.L. Restricted expression of G86R Cu/Zn superoxide dismutase in astrocytes results in astrocytosis but does not cause motoneuron degeneration. *J. Neurosci.* **2000**, *20*, 660–665. [CrossRef] [PubMed]
6. Nguyen, M.D.; Julien, J.P.; Rivest, S. Induction of proinflammatory molecules in mice with amyotrophic lateral sclerosis: No requirement for proapoptotic interleukin-1beta in neurodegeneration. *Ann. Neurol.* **2001**, *50*, 630–639. [CrossRef] [PubMed]
7. Gowing, G.; Dequen, F.; Soucy, G.; Julien, J.P. Absence of tumor necrosis factor-alpha does not affect motor neuron disease caused by superoxide dismutase 1 mutations. *J. Neurosci.* **2006**, *26*, 11397–11402. [CrossRef] [PubMed]
8. Van Damme, P.; Robberecht, W. Recent advances in motor neuron disease. *Curr. Opin. Neurol.* **2009**, *22*, 486–492. [CrossRef] [PubMed]
9. Sanger, F.; Nicklen, S.; Coulson, A.R. DNA sequencing with chain-terminating inhibitors. *Biotechnology* **1992**, *24*, 104–108. [CrossRef]
10. Jiménez-Escrig, A.; Gobernado, I.; Sánchez-Herranz, A. Secuenciación de genoma completo: Un salto cualitativo en los estudios genéticos. *Rev. Neurol.* **2012**, *54*, 692–698.
11. Sanger, F.; Coulson, A.R. A rapid method for determining sequences in DNA by primed synthesis with DNA polymerase. *J. Mol. Biol.* **1975**, *94*, 441–448. [CrossRef]
12. Unamba, C.I.; Nag, A.; Sharma, R.K. Next Generation Sequencing Technologies: The Doorway to the Unexplored Genomics of Non-Model Plants. *Front. Plant Sci.* **2015**, *6*, 1074. [CrossRef]
13. Ansorge, W.J. Next-generation DNA sequencing techniques. *New Biotechnol.* **2009**, *25*, 195–203. [CrossRef] [PubMed]
14. Diamandis, E.P. Next-generation sequencing: A new revolution in molecular diagnostics? *Clin. Chem.* **2009**, *55*, 2088–2092. [CrossRef] [PubMed]
15. Zhang, J.; Chiodini, R.; Badr, A.; Zhang, G. The impact of next-generation sequencing on genomics. *J. Genet. Genomics Yi Chuan Xue Bao* **2011**, *38*, 95–109. [CrossRef] [PubMed]
16. Bick, D.; Dimmock, D. Whole exome and whole genome sequencing. *Curr. Opin. Pediatr.* **2011**, *23*, 594–600. [CrossRef] [PubMed]
17. Biesecker, L.G.; Shianna, K.V.; Mullikin, J.C. Exome sequencing: The expert view. *Genome Biol.* **2011**, *12*, 128. [CrossRef] [PubMed]
18. Wang, A.; Wang, J.; Liu, Y.; Zhou, Y. Mechanisms of Long Non-Coding RNAs in the Assembly and Plasticity of Neural Circuitry. *Front. Neural Circuits* **2017**, *11*, 76. [CrossRef]

19. Gilissen, C.; Hoischen, A.; Brunner, H.G.; Veltman, J.A. Disease gene identification strategies for exome sequencing. *Eur. J. Hum. Genet.* **2012**, *20*, 490–497. [CrossRef]
20. Chong, J.X.; Buckingham, K.J.; Jhangiani, S.N.; Boehm, C.; Sobreira, N.; Smith, J.D.; Harrell, T.M.; McMillin, M.J.; Wiszniewski, W.; Gambin, T.; et al. The Genetic Basis of Mendelian Phenotypes: Discoveries, Challenges, and Opportunities. *Am. J. Hum. Genet.* **2015**, *97*, 199–215. [CrossRef]
21. Zemojtel, T.; Kohler, S.; Mackenroth, L.; Jager, M.; Hecht, J.; Krawitz, P.; Graul-Neumann, L.; Doelken, S.; Ehmke, N.; Spielmann, M.; et al. Effective diagnosis of genetic disease by computational phenotype analysis of the disease-associated genome. *Sci. Transl. Med.* **2014**, *6*, 252ra123. [CrossRef]
22. Köhler, S.; Doelken, S.C.; Mungall, C.J.; Bauer, S.; Firth, H.V.; Bailleul-Forestier, I.; Black, G.C.; Brown, D.L.; Brudno, M.; Campbell, J.; et al. The Human Phenotype Ontology project: Linking molecular biology and disease through phenotype data. *Nucleic Acids Res.* **2014**, *42*, D966–D974. [CrossRef]
23. Robinson, P.N.; Kohler, S.; Bauer, S.; Seelow, D.; Horn, D.; Mundlos, S. The Human Phenotype Ontology: A tool for annotating and analyzing human hereditary disease. *Am. J. Hum. Genet.* **2008**, *83*, 610–615. [CrossRef] [PubMed]
24. Köhler, S.; Schulz, M.H.; Krawitz, P.; Bauer, S.; Dolken, S.; Ott, C.E.; Mundlos, C.; Horn, D.; Mundlos, S.; Robinson, P.N. Clinical diagnostics in human genetics with semantic similarity searches in ontologies. *Am. J. Hum. Genet.* **2009**, *85*, 457–464. [CrossRef] [PubMed]
25. Sifrim, A.; Popovic, D.; Tranchevent, L.C.; Ardeshirdavani, A.; Sakai, R.; Konings, P.; Vermeesch, J.R.; Aerts, J.; De Moor, B.; Moreau, Y. eXtasy: Variant prioritization by genomic data fusion. *Nat. Methods* **2013**, *10*, 1083–1084. [CrossRef] [PubMed]
26. Bauer, S.; Kohler, S.; Schulz, M.H.; Robinson, P.N. Bayesian ontology querying for accurate and noise-tolerant semantic searches. *Bioinformatics* **2012**, *28*, 2502–2508. [CrossRef] [PubMed]
27. Doelken, S.C.; Kohler, S.; Mungall, C.J.; Gkoutos, G.V.; Ruef, B.J.; Smith, C.; Smedley, D.; Bauer, S.; Klopocki, E.; Schofield, P.N.; et al. Phenotypic overlap in the contribution of individual genes to CNV pathogenicity revealed by cross-species computational analysis of single-gene mutations in humans, mice and zebrafish. *Dis. Models Mech.* **2013**, *6*, 358–372. [CrossRef] [PubMed]
28. Al-Qattan, M.M.; Al Abdulkareem, I.; Al Haidan, Y.; Al Balwi, M. A novel mutation in the SHH long-range regulator (ZRS) is associated with preaxial polydactyly, triphalangeal thumb, and severe radial ray deficiency. *Am. J. Med. Genet. Part A* **2012**, *158A*, 2610–2615. [CrossRef] [PubMed]
29. Yang, Y.; Muzny, D.M.; Reid, J.G.; Bainbridge, M.N.; Willis, A.; Ward, P.A.; Braxton, A.; Beuten, J.; Xia, F.; Niu, Z.; et al. Clinical whole-exome sequencing for the diagnosis of mendelian disorders. *N. Engl. J. Med.* **2013**, *369*, 1502–1511. [CrossRef] [PubMed]
30. Van Deerlin, V.M. The genetics and neuropathology of neurodegenerative disorders: Perspectives and implications for research and clinical practice. *Acta Neuropathol.* **2012**, *124*, 297–303. [CrossRef]
31. Ferri, C.P.; Sousa, R.; Albanese, E.; Ribeiro, W.S.; Honyashiki, M. *World Alzheimer Report 2009—Executive Summary*; Alzheimer's Disease International: London, UK, 2009; pp. 1–22.
32. Perrin, R.J.; Fagan, A.M.; Holtzman, D.M. Multimodal techniques for diagnosis and prognosis of Alzheimer's disease. *Nature* **2009**, *461*, 916–922. [CrossRef]
33. Schellenberg, G.D.; Montine, T.J. The genetics and neuropathology of Alzheimer's disease. *Acta Neuropathol.* **2012**, *124*, 305–323. [CrossRef]
34. Gatz, M.; Reynolds, C.A.; Fratiglioni, L.; Johansson, B.; Mortimer, J.A.; Berg, S.; Fiske, A.; Pedersen, N.L. Role of genes and environments for explaining Alzheimer disease. *Arch. Gen. Psychiatry* **2006**, *63*, 168–174. [CrossRef] [PubMed]
35. Kang, J.; Lemaire, H.G.; Unterbeck, A.; Salbaum, J.M.; Masters, C.L.; Grzeschik, K.H.; Multhaup, G.; Beyreuther, K.; Muller-Hill, B. The precursor of Alzheimer's disease amyloid A4 protein resembles a cell-surface receptor. *Nature* **1987**, *325*, 733–736. [CrossRef] [PubMed]
36. Ryman, D.C.; Acosta-Baena, N.; Aisen, P.S.; Bird, T.; Danek, A.; Fox, N.C.; Goate, A.; Frommelt, P.; Ghetti, B.; Langbaum, J.B.; et al. Symptom onset in autosomal dominant Alzheimer disease: A systematic review and meta-analysis. *Neurology* **2014**, *83*, 253–260. [CrossRef] [PubMed]
37. Lopera, F.; Ardilla, A.; Martinez, A.; Madrigal, L.; Arango-Viana, J.C.; Lemere, C.A.; Arango-Lasprilla, J.C.; Hincapie, L.; Arcos-Burgos, M.; Ossa, J.E.; et al. Clinical features of early-onset Alzheimer disease in a large kindred with an E280A presenilin-1 mutation. *JAMA* **1997**, *277*, 793–799. [CrossRef] [PubMed]

38. Lambert, J.C.; Ibrahim-Verbaas, C.A.; Harold, D.; Naj, A.C.; Sims, R.; Bellenguez, C.; DeStafano, A.L.; Bis, J.C.; Beecham, G.W.; Grenier-Boley, B.; et al. Meta-analysis of 74,046 individuals identifies 11 new susceptibility loci for Alzheimer's disease. *Nat. Genet.* **2013**, *45*, 1452–1458. [CrossRef] [PubMed]
39. Jonsson, T.; Stefansson, H.; Steinberg, S.; Jonsdottir, I.; Jonsson, P.V.; Snaedal, J.; Bjornsson, S.; Huttenlocher, J.; Levey, A.I.; Lah, J.J.; et al. Variant of TREM2 associated with the risk of Alzheimer's disease. *N. Engl. J. Med.* **2013**, *368*, 107–116. [CrossRef] [PubMed]
40. Guerreiro, R.; Wojtas, A.; Bras, J.; Carrasquillo, M.; Rogaeva, E.; Majounie, E.; Cruchaga, C.; Sassi, C.; Kauwe, J.S.; Younkin, S.; et al. TREM2 variants in Alzheimer's disease. *N. Engl. J. Med.* **2013**, *368*, 117–127. [CrossRef]
41. Wetzel-Smith, M.K.; Hunkapiller, J.; Bhangale, T.R.; Srinivasan, K.; Maloney, J.A.; Atwal, J.K.; Sa, S.M.; Yaylaoglu, M.B.; Foreman, O.; Ortmann, W.; et al. A rare mutation in UNC5C predisposes to late-onset Alzheimer's disease and increases neuronal cell death. *Nat. Med.* **2014**, *20*, 1452–1457. [CrossRef]
42. Logue, M.W.; Schu, M.; Vardarajan, B.N.; Farrell, J.; Bennett, D.A.; Buxbaum, J.D.; Byrd, G.S.; Ertekin-Taner, N.; Evans, D.; Foroud, T.; et al. Two rare AKAP9 variants are associated with Alzheimer's disease in African Americans. *Alzheimer's Dement. J. Alzheimer's Assoc.* **2014**, *10*, 609–618.e11. [CrossRef]
43. Namba, Y.; Tomonaga, M.; Kawasaki, H.; Otomo, E.; Ikeda, K. Apolipoprotein E immunoreactivity in cerebral amyloid deposits and neurofibrillary tangles in Alzheimer's disease and kuru plaque amyloid in Creutzfeldt-Jakob disease. *Brain Res.* **1991**, *541*, 163–166. [CrossRef]
44. Holtzman, D.M. In vivo effects of ApoE and clusterin on amyloid-beta metabolism and neuropathology. *J. Mol. Neurosci.* **2004**, *23*, 247–254. [CrossRef]
45. Ertekin-Taner, N. Genetics of Alzheimer's disease: A centennial review. *Neurol. Clin.* **2007**, *25*, 611–667. [CrossRef] [PubMed]
46. Sachidanandam, R.; Weissman, D.; Schmidt, S.C.; Kakol, J.M.; Stein, L.D.; Marth, G.; Sherry, S.; Mullikin, J.C.; Mortimore, B.J.; Willey, D.L.; et al. A map of human genome sequence variation containing 1.42 million single nucleotide polymorphisms. *Nature* **2001**, *409*, 928–933. [PubMed]
47. Alzforum. AlzGene—Field Synopsis of Genetic Association Studies in AD. Available online: http://www.alzgene.org/ (accessed on 12 November 2018).
48. Bertram, L.; McQueen, M.B.; Mullin, K.; Blacker, D.; Tanzi, R.E. Systematic meta-analyses of Alzheimer disease genetic association studies: The AlzGene database. *Nat. Genet.* **2007**, *39*, 17–23. [CrossRef] [PubMed]
49. Rogaeva, E.; Meng, Y.; Lee, J.H.; Gu, Y.; Kawarai, T.; Zou, F.; Katayama, T.; Baldwin, C.T.; Cheng, R.; Hasegawa, H.; et al. The neuronal sortilin-related receptor SORL1 is genetically associated with Alzheimer disease. *Nat. Genet.* **2007**, *39*, 168–177. [CrossRef]
50. Dreses-Werringloer, U.; Lambert, J.C.; Vingtdeux, V.; Zhao, H.; Vais, H.; Siebert, A.; Jain, A.; Koppel, J.; Rovelet-Lecrux, A.; Hannequin, D.; et al. A polymorphism in CALHM1 influences Ca^{2+} homeostasis, Abeta levels, and Alzheimer's disease risk. *Cell* **2008**, *133*, 1149–1161. [CrossRef] [PubMed]
51. Lohmueller, K.E.; Pearce, C.L.; Pike, M.; Lander, E.S.; Hirschhorn, J.N. Meta-analysis of genetic association studies supports a contribution of common variants to susceptibility to common disease. *Nat. Genet.* **2003**, *33*, 177–182. [CrossRef] [PubMed]
52. Newton-Cheh, C.; Hirschhorn, J.N. Genetic association studies of complex traits: Design and analysis issues. *Mutat. Res.* **2005**, *573*, 54–69. [CrossRef]
53. Ertekin-Taner, N. Genetics of Alzheimer disease in the pre- and post-GWAS era. *Alzheimer's Res. Ther.* **2010**, *2*, 3. [CrossRef]
54. Grupe, A.; Abraham, R.; Li, Y.; Rowland, C.; Hollingworth, P.; Morgan, A.; Jehu, L.; Segurado, R.; Stone, D.; Schadt, E.; et al. Evidence for novel susceptibility genes for late-onset Alzheimer's disease from a genome-wide association study of putative functional variants. *Hum. Mol. Genet.* **2007**, *16*, 865–873. [CrossRef]
55. Feulner, T.M.; Laws, S.M.; Friedrich, P.; Wagenpfeil, S.; Wurst, S.H.; Riehle, C.; Kuhn, K.A.; Krawczak, M.; Schreiber, S.; Nikolaus, S.; et al. Examination of the current top candidate genes for AD in a genome-wide association study. *Mol. Psychiatry* **2010**, *15*, 756–766. [CrossRef] [PubMed]
56. Reiman, E.M.; Webster, J.A.; Myers, A.J.; Hardy, J.; Dunckley, T.; Zismann, V.L.; Joshipura, K.D.; Pearson, J.V.; Hu-Lince, D.; Huentelman, M.J.; et al. GAB2 alleles modify Alzheimer's risk in APOE epsilon4 carriers. *Neuron* **2007**, *54*, 713–720. [CrossRef] [PubMed]

57. Li, H.; Wetten, S.; Li, L.; St Jean, P.L.; Upmanyu, R.; Surh, L.; Hosford, D.; Barnes, M.R.; Briley, J.D.; Borrie, M.; et al. Candidate single-nucleotide polymorphisms from a genomewide association study of Alzheimer disease. *Arch. Neurol.* **2008**, *65*, 45–53. [CrossRef] [PubMed]
58. Abraham, R.; Moskvina, V.; Sims, R.; Hollingworth, P.; Morgan, A.; Georgieva, L.; Dowzell, K.; Cichon, S.; Hillmer, A.M.; O'Donovan, M.C.; et al. A genome-wide association study for late-onset Alzheimer's disease using DNA pooling. *BMC Med. Genomics* **2008**, *1*, 44. [CrossRef] [PubMed]
59. Carrasquillo, M.M.; Zou, F.; Pankratz, V.S.; Wilcox, S.L.; Ma, L.; Walker, L.P.; Younkin, S.G.; Younkin, C.S.; Younkin, L.H.; Bisceglio, G.D.; et al. Genetic variation in PCDH11X is associated with susceptibility to late-onset Alzheimer's disease. *Nat. Genet.* **2009**, *41*, 192–198. [CrossRef] [PubMed]
60. Poduslo, S.E.; Huang, R.; Huang, J.; Smith, S. Genome screen of late-onset Alzheimer's extended pedigrees identifies TRPC4AP by haplotype analysis. *Am. J. Med. Genet. Part B Neuropsychiatr. Genet.* **2009**, *150*, 50–55. [CrossRef]
61. Harold, D.; Abraham, R.; Hollingworth, P.; Sims, R.; Gerrish, A.; Hamshere, M.L.; Pahwa, J.S.; Moskvina, V.; Dowzell, K.; Williams, A.; et al. Genome-wide association study identifies variants at CLU and PICALM associated with Alzheimer's disease. *Nat. Genet.* **2009**, *41*, 1088–1093. [CrossRef]
62. Lambert, J.C.; Heath, S.; Even, G.; Campion, D.; Sleegers, K.; Hiltunen, M.; Combarros, O.; Zelenika, D.; Bullido, M.J.; Tavernier, B.; et al. Genome-wide association study identifies variants at CLU and CR1 associated with Alzheimer's disease. *Nat. Genet.* **2009**, *41*, 1094–1099. [CrossRef]
63. Coon, K.D.; Myers, A.J.; Craig, D.W.; Webster, J.A.; Pearson, J.V.; Lince, D.H.; Zismann, V.L.; Beach, T.G.; Leung, D.; Bryden, L.; et al. A high-density whole-genome association study reveals that APOE is the major susceptibility gene for sporadic late-onset Alzheimer's disease. *J. Clin. Psychiatry* **2007**, *68*, 613–618. [CrossRef]
64. Genin, E.; Hannequin, D.; Wallon, D.; Sleegers, K.; Hiltunen, M.; Combarros, O.; Bullido, M.J.; Engelborghs, S.; De Deyn, P.; Berr, C.; et al. APOE and Alzheimer disease: A major gene with semi-dominant inheritance. *Mol. Psychiatry* **2011**, *16*, 903–907. [CrossRef]
65. Chen, S.; Parmigiani, G. Meta-analysis of BRCA1 and BRCA2 penetrance. *J. Clin. Oncol.* **2007**, *25*, 1329–1333. [CrossRef] [PubMed]
66. Hadano, S.; Hand, C.K.; Osuga, H.; Yanagisawa, Y.; Otomo, A.; Devon, R.S.; Miyamoto, N.; Showguchi-Miyata, J.; Okada, Y.; Singaraja, R.; et al. A gene encoding a putative GTPase regulator is mutated in familial amyotrophic lateral sclerosis 2. *Nat. Genet.* **2001**, *29*, 166–173. [CrossRef] [PubMed]
67. Burgunder, J.M.; Schols, L.; Baets, J.; Andersen, P.; Gasser, T.; Szolnoki, Z.; Fontaine, B.; Van Broeckhoven, C.; Di Donato, S.; De Jonghe, P.; et al. EFNS guidelines for the molecular diagnosis of neurogenetic disorders: Motoneuron, peripheral nerve and muscle disorders. *Eur. J. Neurol.* **2011**, *18*, 207–217. [CrossRef] [PubMed]
68. Yang, J.; Benyamin, B.; McEvoy, B.P.; Gordon, S.; Henders, A.K.; Nyholt, D.R.; Madden, P.A.; Heath, A.C.; Martin, N.G.; Montgomery, G.W.; et al. Common SNPs explain a large proportion of the heritability for human height. *Nat. Genet.* **2010**, *42*, 565–569. [CrossRef] [PubMed]
69. Yang, J.; Manolio, T.A.; Pasquale, L.R.; Boerwinkle, E.; Caporaso, N.; Cunningham, J.M.; de Andrade, M.; Feenstra, B.; Feingold, E.; Hayes, M.G.; et al. Genome partitioning of genetic variation for complex traits using common SNPs. *Nat. Genet.* **2011**, *43*, 519–525. [CrossRef] [PubMed]
70. Yang, J.; Lee, S.H.; Goddard, M.E.; Visscher, P.M. Genome-wide complex trait analysis (GCTA): Methods, data analyses, and interpretations. *Methods Mol. Biol.* **2013**, *1019*, 215–236. [PubMed]
71. Al-Chalabi, A.; Fang, F.; Hanby, M.F.; Leigh, P.N.; Shaw, C.E.; Ye, W.; Rijsdijk, F. An estimate of amyotrophic lateral sclerosis heritability using twin data. *J. Neurol. Neurosurg. Psychiatry* **2010**, *81*, 1324–1326. [CrossRef]
72. Johnson, J.O.; Mandrioli, J.; Benatar, M.; Abramzon, Y.; Van Deerlin, V.M.; Trojanowski, J.Q.; Gibbs, J.R.; Brunetti, M.; Gronka, S.; Wuu, J.; et al. Exome sequencing reveals VCP mutations as a cause of familial ALS. *Neuron* **2010**, *68*, 857–864. [CrossRef]
73. Byrne, S.; Hardiman, O. Familial aggregation in amyotrophic lateral sclerosis. *Ann. Neurol.* **2010**, *67*, 554. [CrossRef]
74. Huisman, M.H.; de Jong, S.W.; Verwijs, M.C.; Schelhaas, H.J.; van der Kooi, A.J.; de Visser, M.; Veldink, J.H.; van den Berg, L.H. Family history of neurodegenerative and vascular diseases in ALS: A population-based study. *Neurology* **2011**, *77*, 1363–1369. [CrossRef]

75. Johnston, C.A.; Stanton, B.R.; Turner, M.R.; Gray, R.; Blunt, A.H.; Butt, D.; Ampong, M.A.; Shaw, C.E.; Leigh, P.N.; Al-Chalabi, A. Amyotrophic lateral sclerosis in an urban setting: A population based study of inner city London. *J. Neurol.* **2006**, *253*, 1642–1643. [CrossRef] [PubMed]
76. Al-Chalabi, A.; Jones, A.; Troakes, C.; King, A.; Al-Sarraj, S.; van den Berg, L.H. The genetics and neuropathology of amyotrophic lateral sclerosis. *Acta Neuropathol.* **2012**, *124*, 339–352. [CrossRef] [PubMed]
77. Keller, M.F.; Ferrucci, L.; Singleton, A.B.; Tienari, P.J.; Laaksovirta, H.; Restagno, G.; Chio, A.; Traynor, B.J.; Nalls, M.A. Genome-wide analysis of the heritability of amyotrophic lateral sclerosis. *JAMA Neurol.* **2014**, *71*, 1123–1134. [CrossRef] [PubMed]
78. Neumann, M.; Sampathu, D.M.; Kwong, L.K.; Truax, A.C.; Micsenyi, M.C.; Chou, T.T.; Bruce, J.; Schuck, T.; Grossman, M.; Clark, C.M.; et al. Ubiquitinated TDP-43 in frontotemporal lobar degeneration and amyotrophic lateral sclerosis. *Science* **2006**, *314*, 130–133. [CrossRef] [PubMed]
79. Beckman, J.S.; Carson, M.; Smith, C.D.; Koppenol, W.H. ALS, SOD and peroxynitrite. *Nature* **1993**, *364*, 584. [CrossRef]
80. Bosco, D.A.; Morfini, G.; Karabacak, N.M.; Song, Y.; Gros-Louis, F.; Pasinelli, P.; Goolsby, H.; Fontaine, B.A.; Lemay, N.; McKenna-Yasek, D.; et al. Wild-type and mutant SOD1 share an aberrant conformation and a common pathogenic pathway in ALS. *Nat. Neurosci.* **2010**, *13*, 1396–1403. [CrossRef] [PubMed]
81. Crow, J.P.; Sampson, J.B.; Zhuang, Y.; Thompson, J.A.; Beckman, J.S. Decreased zinc affinity of amyotrophic lateral sclerosis-associated superoxide dismutase mutants leads to enhanced catalysis of tyrosine nitration by peroxynitrite. *J. Neurochem.* **1997**, *69*, 1936–1944. [CrossRef] [PubMed]
82. Higgins, C.M.; Jung, C.; Ding, H.; Xu, Z. Mutant Cu, Zn superoxide dismutase that causes motoneuron degeneration is present in mitochondria in the CNS. *J. Neurosci.* **2002**, *22*, RC215. [CrossRef] [PubMed]
83. Ligon, L.A.; LaMonte, B.H.; Wallace, K.E.; Weber, N.; Kalb, R.G.; Holzbaur, E.L. Mutant superoxide dismutase disrupts cytoplasmic dynein in motor neurons. *Neuroreport* **2005**, *16*, 533–536. [CrossRef]
84. Spreux-Varoquaux, O.; Bensimon, G.; Lacomblez, L.; Salachas, F.; Pradat, P.F.; Le Forestier, N.; Marouan, A.; Dib, M.; Meininger, V. Glutamate levels in cerebrospinal fluid in amyotrophic lateral sclerosis: A reappraisal using a new HPLC method with coulometric detection in a large cohort of patients. *J. Neurol. Sci.* **2002**, *193*, 73–78. [CrossRef]
85. Wiedau-Pazos, M.; Goto, J.J.; Rabizadeh, S.; Gralla, E.B.; Roe, J.A.; Lee, M.K.; Valentine, J.S.; Bredesen, D.E. Altered reactivity of superoxide dismutase in familial amyotrophic lateral sclerosis. *Science* **1996**, *271*, 515–518. [CrossRef] [PubMed]
86. Van Deerlin, V.M.; Leverenz, J.B.; Bekris, L.M.; Bird, T.D.; Yuan, W.; Elman, L.B.; Clay, D.; Wood, E.M.; Chen-Plotkin, A.S.; Martinez-Lage, M.; et al. TARDBP mutations in amyotrophic lateral sclerosis with TDP-43 neuropathology: A genetic and histopathological analysis. *Lancet Neurol.* **2008**, *7*, 409–416. [CrossRef]
87. Yokoseki, A.; Shiga, A.; Tan, C.F.; Tagawa, A.; Kaneko, H.; Koyama, A.; Eguchi, H.; Tsujino, A.; Ikeuchi, T.; Kakita, A.; et al. TDP-43 mutation in familial amyotrophic lateral sclerosis. *Ann. Neurol.* **2008**, *63*, 538–542. [CrossRef] [PubMed]
88. Kwiatkowski, T.J., Jr.; Bosco, D.A.; Leclerc, A.L.; Tamrazian, E.; Vanderburg, C.R.; Russ, C.; Davis, A.; Gilchrist, J.; Kasarskis, E.J.; Munsat, T.; et al. Mutations in the FUS/TLS gene on chromosome 16 cause familial amyotrophic lateral sclerosis. *Science* **2009**, *323*, 1205–1208. [CrossRef] [PubMed]
89. Vance, C.; Rogelj, B.; Hortobagyi, T.; De Vos, K.J.; Nishimura, A.L.; Sreedharan, J.; Hu, X.; Smith, B.; Ruddy, D.; Wright, P.; et al. Mutations in FUS, an RNA processing protein, cause familial amyotrophic lateral sclerosis type 6. *Science* **2009**, *323*, 1208–1211. [CrossRef] [PubMed]
90. Deng, H.X.; Chen, W.; Hong, S.T.; Boycott, K.M.; Gorrie, G.H.; Siddique, N.; Yang, Y.; Fecto, F.; Shi, Y.; Zhai, H.; et al. Mutations in UBQLN2 cause dominant X-linked juvenile and adult-onset ALS and ALS/dementia. *Nature* **2011**, *477*, 211–215. [CrossRef] [PubMed]
91. Lansbury, P.T.; Lashuel, H.A. A century-old debate on protein aggregation and neurodegeneration enters the clinic. *Nature* **2006**, *443*, 774–779. [CrossRef] [PubMed]
92. Leigh, P.N.; Whitwell, H.; Garofalo, O.; Buller, J.; Swash, M.; Martin, J.E.; Gallo, J.M.; Weller, R.O.; Anderton, B.H. Ubiquitin-immunoreactive intraneuronal inclusions in amyotrophic lateral sclerosis. Morphology, distribution, and specificity. *Brain A J. Neurol.* **1991**, *114*, 775–788. [CrossRef]
93. Ticozzi, N.; Vance, C.; Leclerc, A.L.; Keagle, P.; Glass, J.D.; McKenna-Yasek, D.; Sapp, P.C.; Silani, V.; Bosco, D.A.; Shaw, C.E.; et al. Mutational analysis reveals the FUS homolog TAF15 as a candidate gene for

familial amyotrophic lateral sclerosis. *Am. J. Med. Genet. Part B Neuropsychiatr. Genet. Off. Publ. Int. Soc. Psychiatr. Genet.* **2011**, *156B*, 285–290. [CrossRef] [PubMed]
94. Lill, C.M.; Abel, O.; Bertram, L.; Al-Chalabi, A. Keeping up with genetic discoveries in amyotrophic lateral sclerosis: The ALSoD and ALSGene databases. *Amyotroph. Lateral Scler. Off. Publ. World Fed. Neurol. Res. Group Motor Neuron Dis.* **2011**, *12*, 238–249. [CrossRef] [PubMed]
95. Goodall, E.F.; Greenway, M.J.; van Marion, I.; Carroll, C.B.; Hardiman, O.; Morrison, K.E. Association of the H63D polymorphism in the hemochromatosis gene with sporadic ALS. *Neurology* **2005**, *65*, 934–937. [CrossRef] [PubMed]
96. Sutedja, N.A.; Sinke, R.J.; Van Vught, P.W.; Van der Linden, M.W.; Wokke, J.H.; Van Duijn, C.M.; Njajou, O.T.; Van der Schouw, Y.T.; Veldink, J.H.; Van den Berg, L.H. The association between H63D mutations in HFE and amyotrophic lateral sclerosis in a Dutch population. *Arch. Neurol.* **2007**, *64*, 63–67. [CrossRef] [PubMed]
97. Praline, J.; Blasco, H.; Vourc'h, P.; Rat, V.; Gendrot, C.; Camu, W.; Andres, C.R. Study of the HFE gene common polymorphisms in French patients with sporadic amyotrophic lateral sclerosis. *J. Neurol. Sci.* **2012**, *317*, 58–61. [CrossRef] [PubMed]
98. Greenway, M.J.; Andersen, P.M.; Russ, C.; Ennis, S.; Cashman, S.; Donaghy, C.; Patterson, V.; Swingler, R.; Kieran, D.; Prehn, J.; et al. ANG mutations segregate with familial and 'sporadic' amyotrophic lateral sclerosis. *Nat. Genet.* **2006**, *38*, 411–413. [CrossRef] [PubMed]
99. Rooke, K.; Figlewicz, D.A.; Han, F.Y.; Rouleau, G.A. Analysis of the KSP repeat of the neurofilament heavy subunit in familiar amyotrophic lateral sclerosis. *Neurology* **1996**, *46*, 789–790. [CrossRef] [PubMed]
100. Couthouis, J.; Hart, M.P.; Erion, R.; King, O.D.; Diaz, Z.; Nakaya, T.; Ibrahim, F.; Kim, H.J.; Mojsilovic-Petrovic, J.; Panossian, S.; et al. Evaluating the role of the FUS/TLS-related gene EWSR1 in amyotrophic lateral sclerosis. *Hum. Mol. Genet.* **2012**, *21*, 2899–2911. [CrossRef] [PubMed]
101. Couthouis, J.; Hart, M.P.; Shorter, J.; DeJesus-Hernandez, M.; Erion, R.; Oristano, R.; Liu, A.X.; Ramos, D.; Jethava, N.; Hosangadi, D.; et al. A yeast functional screen predicts new candidate ALS disease genes. *Proc. Natl. Acad. Sci. USA* **2011**, *108*, 20881–20890. [CrossRef]
102. Shatunov, A.; Mok, K.; Newhouse, S.; Weale, M.E.; Smith, B.; Vance, C.; Johnson, L.; Veldink, J.H.; van Es, M.A.; van den Berg, L.H.; et al. Chromosome 9p21 in sporadic amyotrophic lateral sclerosis in the UK and seven other countries: A genome-wide association study. *Lancet Neurol.* **2010**, *9*, 986–994. [CrossRef]
103. van Rheenen, W.; Shatunov, A.; Dekker, A.M.; McLaughlin, R.L.; Diekstra, F.P.; Pulit, S.L.; van der Spek, R.A.; Vosa, U.; de Jong, S.; Robinson, M.R.; et al. Genome-wide association analyses identify new risk variants and the genetic architecture of amyotrophic lateral sclerosis. *Nat. Genet.* **2016**, *48*, 1043–1048. [CrossRef]
104. Cirulli, E.T.; Lasseigne, B.N.; Petrovski, S.; Sapp, P.C.; Dion, P.A.; Leblond, C.S.; Couthouis, J.; Lu, Y.F.; Wang, Q.; Krueger, B.J.; et al. Exome sequencing in amyotrophic lateral sclerosis identifies risk genes and pathways. *Science* **2015**, *347*, 1436–1441. [CrossRef]
105. Ferraiuolo, L.; Kirby, J.; Grierson, A.J.; Sendtner, M.; Shaw, P.J. Molecular pathways of motor neuron injury in amyotrophic lateral sclerosis. *Nat. Rev. Neurol.* **2011**, *7*, 616–630. [CrossRef]
106. Vucic, S.; Kiernan, M.C. Cortical excitability testing distinguishes Kennedy's disease from amyotrophic lateral sclerosis. *Clin. Neurophysiol.* **2008**, *119*, 1088–1096. [CrossRef]
107. Rothstein, J.D.; Martin, L.J.; Kuncl, R.W. Decreased glutamate transport by the brain and spinal cord in amyotrophic lateral sclerosis. *N. Engl. J. Med.* **1992**, *326*, 1464–1468. [CrossRef] [PubMed]
108. Winkler, E.A.; Sengillo, J.D.; Sagare, A.P.; Zhao, Z.; Ma, Q.; Zuniga, E.; Wang, Y.; Zhong, Z.; Sullivan, J.S.; Griffin, J.H.; et al. Blood-spinal cord barrier disruption contributes to early motor-neuron degeneration in ALS-model mice. *Proc. Natl. Acad. Sci. USA* **2014**, *111*, E1035–E1042. [CrossRef] [PubMed]
109. Liu, J.; Lillo, C.; Jonsson, P.A.; Vande Velde, C.; Ward, C.M.; Miller, T.M.; Subramaniam, J.R.; Rothstein, J.D.; Marklund, S.; Andersen, P.M.; et al. Toxicity of familial ALS-linked SOD1 mutants from selective recruitment to spinal mitochondria. *Neuron* **2004**, *43*, 5–17. [CrossRef] [PubMed]
110. Vande Velde, C.; Miller, T.M.; Cashman, N.R.; Cleveland, D.W. Selective association of misfolded ALS-linked mutant SOD1 with the cytoplasmic face of mitochondria. *Proc. Natl. Acad. Sci. USA* **2008**, *105*, 4022–4027. [CrossRef]
111. Sathasivam, S.; Grierson, A.J.; Shaw, P.J. Characterization of the caspase cascade in a cell culture model of SOD1-related familial amyotrophic lateral sclerosis: Expression, activation and therapeutic effects of inhibition. *Neuropathol. Appl. Neurobiol.* **2005**, *31*, 467–485. [CrossRef]

112. Sathasivam, S.; Shaw, P.J. Apoptosis in amyotrophic lateral sclerosis–what is the evidence? *Lancet Neurol.* **2005**, *4*, 500–509. [CrossRef]
113. Wiedemann, F.R.; Manfredi, G.; Mawrin, C.; Beal, M.F.; Schon, E.A. Mitochondrial DNA and respiratory chain function in spinal cords of ALS patients. *J. Neurochem.* **2002**, *80*, 616–625. [CrossRef]
114. Blackburn, D.; Sargsyan, S.; Monk, P.N.; Shaw, P.J. Astrocyte function and role in motor neuron disease: A future therapeutic target? *Glia* **2009**, *57*, 1251–1264. [CrossRef]
115. Duffy, L.M.; Chapman, A.L.; Shaw, P.J.; Grierson, A.J. Review: The role of mitochondria in the pathogenesis of amyotrophic lateral sclerosis. *Neuropathol. Appl. Neurobiol.* **2011**, *37*, 336–352. [CrossRef] [PubMed]
116. Rao, S.D.; Weiss, J.H. Excitotoxic and oxidative cross-talk between motor neurons and glia in ALS pathogenesis. *Trends Neurosci.* **2004**, *27*, 17–23. [CrossRef] [PubMed]
117. Sargsyan, S.A.; Monk, P.N.; Shaw, P.J. Microglia as potential contributors to motor neuron injury in amyotrophic lateral sclerosis. *Glia* **2005**, *51*, 241–253. [CrossRef] [PubMed]
118. Fischer, L.R.; Culver, D.G.; Tennant, P.; Davis, A.A.; Wang, M.; Castellano-Sanchez, A.; Khan, J.; Polak, M.A.; Glass, J.D. Amyotrophic lateral sclerosis is a distal axonopathy: Evidence in mice and man. *Exp. Neurol.* **2004**, *185*, 232–240. [CrossRef]
119. Piao, Y.S.; Wakabayashi, K.; Kakita, A.; Yamada, M.; Hayashi, S.; Morita, T.; Ikuta, F.; Oyanagi, K.; Takahashi, H. Neuropathology with clinical correlations of sporadic amyotrophic lateral sclerosis: 102 autopsy cases examined between 1962 and 2000. *Brain Pathol.* **2003**, *13*, 10–22. [CrossRef] [PubMed]
120. Hooten, K.G.; Beers, D.R.; Zhao, W.; Appel, S.H. Protective and Toxic Neuroinflammation in Amyotrophic Lateral Sclerosis. *Neurother. J. Am. Soc. Exp. Neurother.* **2015**, *12*, 364–375. [CrossRef]
121. Gonzalez, H.; Elgueta, D.; Montoya, A.; Pacheco, R. Neuroimmune regulation of microglial activity involved in neuroinflammation and neurodegenerative diseases. *J. Neuroimmunol.* **2014**, *274*, 1–13. [CrossRef]
122. More, S.V.; Kumar, H.; Kim, I.S.; Song, S.Y.; Choi, D.K. Cellular and molecular mediators of neuroinflammation in the pathogenesis of Parkinson's disease. *Mediat. Inflamm.* **2013**, *2013*, 952375. [CrossRef]
123. Gendelman, H.E.; Appel, S.H. Neuroprotective activities of regulatory T cells. *Trends Mol. Med.* **2011**, *17*, 687–688. [CrossRef]
124. Nicolas, A.; Kenna, K.P.; Renton, A.; Ticozzi, N.; Faghri, F.; Chia, R.; Dominov, J.; Kenna, B.; Nalls, M.A.; Keagle, P.; et al. Genome-wide Analyses Identify KIF5A as a Novel ALS Gene. *Neuron* **2018**, *97*, 1268–1283. [CrossRef]
125. Diekstra, F.P.; van Vught, P.W.; van Rheenen, W.; Koppers, M.; Pasterkamp, R.J.; van Es, M.A.; Schelhaas, H.J.; de Visser, M.; Robberecht, W.; Van Damme, P.; et al. UNC13A is a modifier of survival in amyotrophic lateral sclerosis. *Neurobiol. Aging* **2012**, *33*, 630. [CrossRef] [PubMed]
126. Fogh, I.; Lin, K.; Tiloca, C.; Rooney, J.; Gellera, C.; Diekstra, F.P.; Ratti, A.; Shatunov, A.; van Es, M.A.; Proitsi, P.; et al. Association of a Locus in the CAMTA1 Gene with Survival in Patients with Sporadic Amyotrophic Lateral Sclerosis. *JAMA Neurol.* **2016**, *73*, 812–820. [CrossRef] [PubMed]
127. Lill, C.M.; Rengmark, A.; Pihlstrom, L.; Fogh, I.; Shatunov, A.; Sleiman, P.M.; Wang, L.S.; Liu, T.; Lassen, C.F.; Meissner, E.; et al. The role of TREM2 R47H as a risk factor for Alzheimer's disease, frontotemporal lobar degeneration, amyotrophic lateral sclerosis, and Parkinson's disease. *Alzheimer's Dement. J. Alzheimer's Assoc.* **2015**, *11*, 1407–1416. [CrossRef] [PubMed]
128. Holm, I.E.; Alstrup, A.K.; Luo, Y. Genetically modified pig models for neurodegenerative disorders. *J. Pathol.* **2016**, *238*, 267–287. [CrossRef] [PubMed]
129. Dauer, W.; Przedborski, S. Parkinson's disease: Mechanisms and models. *Neuron* **2003**, *39*, 889–909. [CrossRef]
130. Tieu, K. A guide to neurotoxic animal models of Parkinson's disease. *Cold Spring Harbor Perspect. Med.* **2011**, *1*, a009316. [CrossRef] [PubMed]
131. Ostergaard, K.; Holm, I.E.; Zimmer, J. Tyrosine hydroxylase and acetylcholinesterase in the domestic pig mesencephalon: An immunocytochemical and histochemical study. *J. Comp. Neurol.* **1992**, *322*, 149–166. [CrossRef] [PubMed]
132. Moon, J.H.; Kim, J.H.; Im, H.J.; Lee, D.S.; Park, E.J.; Song, K.; Oh, H.J.; Hyun, S.B.; Kang, S.C.; Kim, H.; et al. Proposed Motor Scoring System in a Porcine Model of Parkinson's Disease induced by Chronic Subcutaneous Injection of MPTP. *Exp. Neurobiol.* **2014**, *23*, 258–265. [CrossRef] [PubMed]

133. Larsen, K.; Bendixen, C. Characterization of the porcine FBX07 gene: The first step towards generation of a pig model for Parkinsonian pyramidal syndrome. *Mol. Biol. Rep.* **2012**, *39*, 1517–1526. [CrossRef]
134. Larsen, K.; Madsen, L.B.; Farajzadeh, L.; Bendixen, C. Splicing variants of porcine synphilin-1. *Meta Gene* **2015**, *5*, 32–42. [CrossRef] [PubMed]
135. Lucking, C.B.; Durr, A.; Bonifati, V.; Vaughan, J.; De Michele, G.; Gasser, T.; Harhangi, B.S.; Meco, G.; Denefle, P.; Wood, N.W.; et al. Association between early-onset Parkinson's disease and mutations in the parkin gene. *N. Engl. J. Med.* **2000**, *342*, 1560–1567. [CrossRef] [PubMed]
136. Pankratz, N.; Pauciulo, M.W.; Elsaesser, V.E.; Marek, D.K.; Halter, C.A.; Wojcieszek, J.; Rudolph, A.; Shults, C.W.; Foroud, T.; Nichols, W.C. Mutations in DJ-1 are rare in familial Parkinson disease. *Neurosci. Lett.* **2006**, *408*, 209–213. [CrossRef] [PubMed]
137. Chartier-Harlin, M.C.; Dachsel, J.C.; Vilarino-Guell, C.; Lincoln, S.J.; Lepretre, F.; Hulihan, M.M.; Kachergus, J.; Milnerwood, A.J.; Tapia, L.; Song, M.S.; et al. Translation initiator EIF4G1 mutations in familial Parkinson disease. *Am. J. Hum. Genet.* **2011**, *89*, 398–406. [CrossRef] [PubMed]
138. Zimprich, A.; Benet-Pages, A.; Struhal, W.; Graf, E.; Eck, S.H.; Offman, M.N.; Haubenberger, D.; Spielberger, S.; Schulte, E.C.; Lichtner, P.; et al. A mutation in VPS35, encoding a subunit of the retromer complex, causes late-onset Parkinson disease. *Am. J. Hum. Genet.* **2011**, *89*, 168–175. [CrossRef] [PubMed]
139. Vilarino-Guell, C.; Wider, C.; Ross, O.A.; Dachsel, J.C.; Kachergus, J.M.; Lincoln, S.J.; Soto-Ortolaza, A.I.; Cobb, S.A.; Wilhoite, G.J.; Bacon, J.A.; et al. VPS35 mutations in Parkinson disease. *Am. J. Hum. Genet.* **2011**, *89*, 162–167. [CrossRef] [PubMed]
140. Foo, J.N.; Liu, J.; Tan, E.K. Next-generation sequencing diagnostics for neurological diseases/disorders: From a clinical perspective. *Hum. Genet.* **2013**, *132*, 721–734. [CrossRef] [PubMed]
141. Houlden, H.; Singleton, A.B. The genetics and neuropathology of Parkinson's disease. *Acta Neuropathol.* **2012**, *124*, 325–338. [CrossRef]
142. Polymeropoulos, M.H.; Lavedan, C.; Leroy, E.; Ide, S.E.; Dehejia, A.; Dutra, A.; Pike, B.; Root, H.; Rubenstein, J.; Boyer, R.; et al. Mutation in the alpha-synuclein gene identified in families with Parkinson's disease. *Science* **1997**, *276*, 2045–2047. [CrossRef]
143. Singleton, A.; Gwinn-Hardy, K. Parkinson's disease and dementia with Lewy bodies: A difference in dose? *Lancet* **2004**, *364*, 1105–1107. [CrossRef]
144. Shimura, H.; Hattori, N.; Kubo, S.; Yoshikawa, M.; Kitada, T.; Matsumine, H.; Asakawa, S.; Minoshima, S.; Yamamura, Y.; Shimizu, N.; et al. Immunohistochemical and subcellular localization of Parkin protein: Absence of protein in autosomal recessive juvenile parkinsonism patients. *Ann. Neurol.* **1999**, *45*, 668–672. [CrossRef]
145. Nagakubo, D.; Taira, T.; Kitaura, H.; Ikeda, M.; Tamai, K.; Iguchi-Ariga, S.M.; Ariga, H. DJ-1, a novel oncogene which transforms mouse NIH3T3 cells in cooperation with ras. *Biochem. Biophys. Res. Commun.* **1997**, *231*, 509–513. [CrossRef] [PubMed]
146. Unoki, M.; Nakamura, Y. Growth-suppressive effects of BPOZ and EGR2, two genes involved in the PTEN signaling pathway. *Oncogene* **2001**, *20*, 4457–4465. [CrossRef] [PubMed]
147. Matsui, M.; Corey, D.R. Non-coding RNAs as drug targets. *Nat. Rev. Drug Discov.* **2017**, *16*, 167–179. [CrossRef] [PubMed]
148. Davidovich, C.; Cech, T.R. The recruitment of chromatin modifiers by long noncoding RNAs: Lessons from PRC2. *RNA* **2015**, *21*, 2007–2022. [CrossRef] [PubMed]
149. Zhao, J.; Sun, B.K.; Erwin, J.A.; Song, J.J.; Lee, J.T. Polycomb proteins targeted by a short repeat RNA to the mouse X chromosome. *Science* **2008**, *322*, 750–756. [CrossRef] [PubMed]
150. Leucci, E.; Vendramin, R.; Spinazzi, M.; Laurette, P.; Fiers, M.; Wouters, J.; Radaelli, E.; Eyckerman, S.; Leonelli, C.; Vanderheyden, K.; et al. Melanoma addiction to the long non-coding RNA SAMMSON. *Nature* **2016**, *531*, 518–522. [CrossRef] [PubMed]
151. Meng, L.; Person, R.E.; Beaudet, A.L. Ube3a-ATS is an atypical RNA polymerase II transcript that represses the paternal expression of Ube3a. *Hum. Mol. Genet.* **2012**, *21*, 3001–3012. [CrossRef]
152. Eissmann, M.; Gutschner, T.; Hammerle, M.; Gunther, S.; Caudron-Herger, M.; Gross, M.; Schirmacher, P.; Rippe, K.; Braun, T.; Zornig, M.; et al. Loss of the abundant nuclear non-coding RNA MALAT1 is compatible with life and development. *RNA Biol.* **2012**, *9*, 1076–1087. [CrossRef]

153. Wang, D.Q.; Fu, P.; Yao, C.; Zhu, L.S.; Hou, T.Y.; Chen, J.G.; Lu, Y.; Liu, D.; Zhu, L.Q. Long Non-coding RNAs, Novel Culprits, or Bodyguards in Neurodegenerative Diseases. *Mol. Ther. Nucleic Acids* **2018**, *10*, 269–276. [CrossRef]
154. Yohe, S.; Thyagarajan, B. Review of Clinical Next-Generation Sequencing. *Arch. Pathol. Lab. Med.* **2017**, *141*, 1544–1557. [CrossRef]
155. Zhu, W.; Zhang, X.Y.; Marjani, S.L.; Zhang, J.; Zhang, W.; Wu, S.; Pan, X. Next-generation molecular diagnosis: Single-cell sequencing from bench to bedside. *Cell. Mol. Life Sci.* **2017**, *74*, 869–880. [CrossRef] [PubMed]
156. Tsai, A.C.; Liu, X. Toward Best Practice in Using Molecular Diagnosis to Guide Medical Management, Are We There Yet? *N. Am. J. Med. Sci.* **2014**, *7*, 199–200.
157. Andersen, P.M.; Abrahams, S.; Borasio, G.D.; de Carvalho, M.; Chio, A.; Van Damme, P.; Hardiman, O.; Kollewe, K.; Morrison, K.E.; Petri, S.; et al. EFNS guidelines on the clinical management of amyotrophic lateral sclerosis (MALS)—revised report of an EFNS task force. *Eur. J. Neurol.* **2012**, *19*, 360–375. [PubMed]

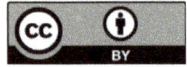

© 2018 by the authors. Licensee MDPI, Basel, Switzerland. This article is an open access article distributed under the terms and conditions of the Creative Commons Attribution (CC BY) license (http://creativecommons.org/licenses/by/4.0/).

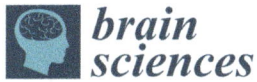

Review

Parkinson's Disease and Metal Storage Disorders: A Systematic Review

Edward Botsford [1,*], Jayan George [2,3] and Ellen E. Buckley [4,5]

1. University of Sheffield Medical School, Beech Hill Road, Sheffield S10 2RX, UK
2. General Surgical Department, Sheffield Teaching Hospitals NHS Foundation Trust, Herries Road, Sheffield S5 7AU, UK; jayan.george@aol.com
3. University of Sheffield, Western Bank, S10 2TN Sheffield, UK
4. Sheffield Institute for Translational Neuroscience, University of Sheffield, 385a Glossop Road, Sheffield S10 2HQ, UK; e.e.buckley@sheffield.ac.uk
5. INSIGNEO Institute for in silico Medicine, University of Sheffield, Pam Liversidge Building, Sheffield S1 3JD, UK
* Correspondence: ebotsford1@sheffield.ac.uk; Tel.: +44-(0)114-222-2272

Received: 9 October 2018; Accepted: 30 October 2018; Published: 31 October 2018

Abstract: Metal storage disorders (MSDs) are a set of rare inherited conditions with variable clinical pictures including neurological dysfunction. The objective of this study was, through a systematic review, to identify the prevalence of Parkinsonism in patients with MSDs in order to uncover novel pathways implemented in Parkinson's disease. Human studies describing patients of any age with an MSD diagnosis were analysed. Foreign language publications as well as animal and cellular studies were excluded. Searches were conducted through PubMed and Ovid between April and September 2018. A total of 53 publications were identified including 43 case reports, nine cross-sectional studies, and one cohort study. The publication year ranged from 1981 to 2018. The most frequently identified MSDs were Pantothenate kinase-associated neurodegeneration (PKAN) with 11 papers describing Parkinsonism, Hereditary hemochromatosis (HH) (7 papers), and Wilson's disease (6 papers). The mean ages of onset of Parkinsonism for these MSDs were 33, 53, and 48 years old, respectively. The Parkinsonian features described in the PKAN and HH patients were invariably atypical while the majority (4/6) of the Wilson's disease papers had a typical picture. This paper has highlighted a relationship between MSDs and Parkinsonism. However, due to the low-level evidence identified, further research is required to better define what the relationship is.

Keywords: Parkinson's disease; Parkinsonism; metal storage disorders; inborn error of metabolism

1. Introduction

Parkinson's disease (PD) is a common and debilitating neurodegenerative disorder. First described in 1817 by James Parkinson, PD is a chronic condition distinguished by bradykinesia, rigidity, postural instability, and resting tremor often described as "pill-rolling." The clinical features are due to the loss of dopaminergic neurones located in the pars compacta of the substantia nigra. Why these neurons are lost is poorly understood. However, numerous studies from animal models and familial cases of PD have identified that accumulation of cytoplasmic inclusions of alpha-synuclein (α-synuclein) called Lewy bodies, oxidative stress, and mitochondrial dysfunction may all play a pathogenic role in their destruction [1,2].

Despite multiple well-documented risk factors suggesting an environmental association such as well-water drinking, pesticide exposure, head injury, and rural living [3], only increased age carries sufficient statistical evidence to be causative [4]. Male gender and Caucasian ethnicity were reported to increase the risk of PD in research studies while tobacco smoking has been found to be protective. Therefore, the existence of other aetiological mechanisms not yet identified must be considered.

Parkinsonism is a clinical picture of a tremor, rigidity, bradykinesia, and postural instability most frequently caused by sporadic PD. However, it has been described in many other conditions. Parkinsonism can be associated with additional features such as dystonia, early autonomic dysfunction, a rapidly progressive disease course, or levodopa unresponsiveness [5]. In this instance, it is described as atypical Parkinsonism since it differs from the typical clinical picture seen in Parkinson's disease.

Inborn errors of metabolism (IEMs) are a large collection of individually rare but collectively common inherited conditions [6]. They are a diverse set of conditions that occur as a result of a monogenic mutation resulting in a deficiency of an enzyme or cofactor [7]. Metal storage disorders are a large subset of these.

Studies have found that patients with PD have increased levels of iron accumulation in the basal ganglia compared with healthy controls [8]. Research has also been conducted into the potential toxic mechanisms of iron causing nigral cell death and leading to PD features in sporadic PD patients even though it remains unclear whether neuronal death is a direct result of iron accumulation or if the accumulation is a by-product of dopaminergic cell death [9].

This systematic review aims to identify whether there is a wider pathological link between PD and metal storage disorders by exploring published accounts of Parkinsonism in patients with a previously diagnosed metal storage disorder. Identifying other conditions that produce Parkinsonian-like clinical features may uncover novel pathological mechanisms that contribute to the development of PD. In addition, this paper will discuss whether the clinical features seen in the patients with metal storage disorders displaying Parkinsonism are of a typical picture seen in PD or if they are more similar to atypical Parkinsonism.

2. Materials and Methods

This systematic review was conducted by following the Preferred Reporting Items for Systematic Reviews and Meta-Analyses (PRISMA) 2009 guidance [10].

2.1. Search Terms

Systematic literature searches were conducted in the PubMed and Ovid SP databases including all published articles prior to the search date. The last search was completed on 6 September, 2018. The titles and abstracts were searched by combining two search terms (Term A and Term B). Term A was 'Parkinson,' 'Parkinson's,' 'Parkinsonism,' or 'Parkinsonian' while Term B included each of the individual metal storage disorders. A list of metal storage disorders was collated from a relevant review article [11]. A full list of the search terms can be found in Appendix A.

2.2. Inclusion Criteria

Human studies of all designs were considered except review articles. Only publications describing patients with a definite genomic or biochemical diagnosis of a metal storage disorder were analysed. Publications reporting adults, children, and infants were all included since metal storage disorders and Parkinsonian features can present at any age. Cohorts from all nationalities and ethnic backgrounds were also included.

2.3. Exclusion Criteria

Animal and cellular model studies were excluded as well as autopsy reports. Papers describing PD patients with MSD associated gene mutations were also excluded unless they had a confirmed diagnosis of that disorder. Publications written in languages other than English, without whole text translations available, were excluded. Reviews and letters to editors were also excluded but the references examined to identify any potentially relevant references that the searches had omitted were accepted.

2.4. Selection Process

The publications acquired from the searches were screened in line with the selection criteria by reading the titles and abstracts to assess relevance. Afterward, full texts were sought for all papers eligible for inclusion. Two reviewers conducted this screening process to ensure adherence to selection criteria. Conflicts were resolved through discussion between the reviewers.

2.5. Data Extraction

The primary outcomes extracted from the publications were the type of study, the IEM affecting the patients reported in the study, and whether the patient had features of typical or atypical Parkinsonism. Patients were identified as possessing atypical Parkinsonism if there was evidence of early autonomic dysfunction, a rapidly progressive course, lack of asymmetrical features at onset, and a poor response to conventional levodopa therapy or a Parkinson-Plus syndrome, as per the definition in the introduction. Where available, the gender, age of onset of Parkinsonian features, smoking status, and ethnicity were recorded as secondary outcomes. A breakdown of the data collected from each individual paper including the clinical picture of the patients can be found in Table A1.

3. Results

In total, 967 publications were identified corresponding to 827 unique articles which underwent the screening process. Following the title and abstract review, 730 were excluded since they did not satisfy the inclusion criteria. Following full text screening, a further 53 records were excluded. Six additional relevant publications were identified from hand searching the reference lists of the reviews and letters identified in the searches. A total of 50 papers were included in this review. Figure 1 shows a PRISMA flowchart of the selection process. The final group of articles consisted of 40 (80.0%) case reports and series, nine (18.0%) cross-sectional studies, and one (2.0%) cohort study (Table 1). The year of publications ranged from 1981 to 2018 with three (6.0%) papers published before 1990, three (6.0%) papers published in the decade between 1991 to 2000, 12 (24.0%) papers published from 2001 to 2010, and 32 (64.0%) papers published in the current decade from 2011 to 2018 (Table 1).

Table 1. Characteristics of included publications.

Year of Publication Range	1981–2018
Number of Publications per Decade	
Before 1990	3
1991–2000	3
2001–2010	12
2011–2018	32
Type of Study	
Cohort study	1
Cross-sectional study	9
Case reports/series	40

Typical Parkinsonism was reported in 16 (32.0%) publications and atypical in 38 (76.0%) publications, which is shown in Table 2. Of these papers, four described subjects with both typical and atypical features. Additionally, 173 patients were reported to have Parkinsonism, 86 (49.7%) were male, and the average age of onset was 35 years old. The ratio of males to females observed was 0.99:1 (86 males to 87 females). The smoking status was not reported in any of the publications (Appendix B).

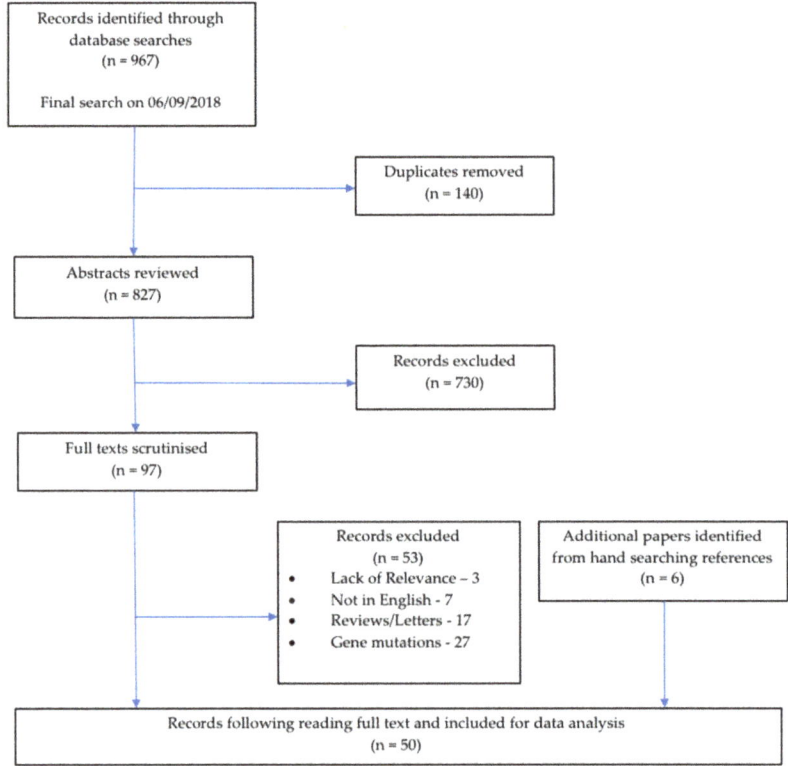

Figure 1. Prisma flow chart illustrating the search strategy and the selection process.

Pantothenate kinase-associated neurodegeneration (PKAN), which is the most prevalent neurodegenerative brain iron accumulation (NBIA) disorder, was the most documented metal storage disorder and was reported in 11 papers. All of these publications described patients displaying features of atypical Parkinsonism. Three papers also described subjects with typical Parkinsonian features. Within the 85 PKAN patients reflected by these articles, the mean age of onset of Parkinsonism was 33 years old. The gender ratio was 1.36:1 with 49 males and 36 females described. PLA2G6-associated neurodegeneration (PLAN) was another frequently identified NBIA with three publications identified. Typical parkinsonism features were described by two of these papers while the remaining publications reported atypical Parkinsonism. Other NBIAs identified beta-propeller protein-associated neurodegeneration (BPAN) with five publications (four with atypical Parkinsonism and one with typical features), Kufor-Rakeb Syndrome with five articles (all atypical, although one described patients with typical features), and mitochondrial-membrane protein-associated neurodegeneration (MPAN) (three papers describing atypical parkinsonism). In addition, three publications described atypical features in subjects with neuroferritinopathy and one paper described a patient with Aceruloplasminemia presenting with features of atypical Parkinsonism. An additional paper described a subject with atypical features who suffered from an unknown type of NBIA.

Table 2. Characteristics of the disorder-related parkinsonism described in the included publications, in order of the number of papers identified.

Condition	Metal Involved	Brain Region Implicated	Total No. of Papers (No. Typical, No. Atypical)	No. (% Total) of Male and Female Patients Described	Average Age of Patients (Years, Mean ± Standard Error)
Panthonase Kinase associated Neurodegeneration (PKAN)	Iron	Basal ganglia (GP, SN)	11 (3;11)	49 M (57.6%) 36 F (42.4%)	33 ± 3.8
Hereditary Haemochromatosis	Iron	-	7 (4;3)	10 M (71.4%) 4 F (28.6%)	53 ± 3.3
Wilson's Disease	Copper	Basal ganglia (PMN, GP)	6 (6;4)	3 M (33.3%) 6 F (66.6%)	46 ± 6.8
Beta-Propeller Protein-Associated Neurodegeneration (BPAN)	Iron	Basal ganglia (SN, GP)	5 (1,4)	3 M (9.7%) 28 F (90.3%)	27 ± 1.1
Kufor-Rakeb Syndrome	Iron	Basal Ganglia (SN, GP)	5 (1;5)	10 M (90.9%) 1 F (9.1%)	13 ± 0.7
Mitochondrial-Membrane Protein-Associated Neurodegeneration (MPAN)	Iron	Basal Ganglia (SN, GP)	3 (0;3)	1 M (50.0%) 1 F (50.0%)	25 ± 10.0
Neuroferritinopathy	Iron	Cerebellum, Basal ganglia, motor cortex	3 (0;3)	5 F (100.0%)	61 ± 17.5
PLA2G6-Associated Neurodegeneration (PLAN)	Iron	Basal ganglia (SN, GP)	3 (2;1)	3 M (60.0%) 2 F (40.0%)	24 ± 5.2
Pseudohypoparathyroidism	Calcium	Basal ganglia, deep white matter	3 (0;3)	1 M (33.3%) 2 F (66.6%)	43 ± 11.8
Fahr Disease	Calcium	Basal ganglia, deep white matter, cerebellum	2 (1;1)	1 M (50.0%) 1 F (50.0%)	56 ± 6.0
Aceruloplasminemia	Iron	Basal ganglia	1 (0;1)	4 M (80.0%) 1 F (20.0%)	NA
Neurodegenerative Brain Iron Accumulation (NBIA), Unknown Type	Iron	-	1 (0;1)	1 M (100.0%)	73 ± 0.0
Total	-	-	50 (16;38)	86 M (49.7%) 87 F (50.3%)	35 ± 1.6

GP = Globus Pallidus, F = Female, M = Male, PMN = Putamen, SN = Substantia Nigra, NA = Not Available.

After PKAN and NBIAs, the next most reported metal storage disorders were Hereditary Haemochromatosis (HH) and Wilson's disease. Seven articles were identified that reported patients with HH and four papers (57.1%) described typical Parkinsonism. In these publications, 14 subjects were described including 10 males and 4 females (a ratio of 2.5:1). The mean age of onset of Parkinsonism in these patients was calculated at 53 years of age. Parkinsonism in Wilson's disease patients was reported in six papers in which four (66.6%) described typical features while the remaining two papers (33.3%) displayed atypical pictures. The mean age of onset in the patients described was 46 years of age and a gender ratio 0.75:1 (three males and six females).

4. Discussion

Parkinsonian presentation in patients with metal storage disorders is an area of growing interest. The number of publications identified in this study increases each decade. While only three articles were published earlier than 1990, between the years 2010 to 2018, 29 papers were identified. This demonstrates an increasing amount of research being conducted in this field and a growing appreciation for a possible correlation between Parkinsonism and metal storage disorders.

The family of neurodegenerative brain iron accumulation (NBIA) disorders includes Pantothenate kinase-associated neurodegeneration (PKAN), Aceruloplasminemia, beta-propeller protein-associated neurodegeneration (BPAN), Kufor-Rakeb Syndrome, mitochondrial-membrane protein-associated neurodegeneration (MPAN), neuroferritinopathy, and PLA2G6-associated neurodegeneration (PLAN). Articles discussing all of these disorders were identified by our searches and described patients displaying Parkinsonism. These all showed a similar phenotype with young average ages of onset of Parkinsonism ranging from 13 years old (Kufor-Rakeb syndrome) to 61 years old (neuroferritinopathy) and predominantly atypical Parkinsonian features. This reflects the similar pathologies across the NBIA family of disorders. In all NBIAs, increased deposition of iron in brain tissue is observed. It is unclear whether this deposition is the direct cause of neurodegeneration or if it is simply a marker of the degeneration occurring as a result of some other pathological mechanism. However, Parkinsonism as well as dystonia appears well documented across all NBIAs.

In line with our findings, PKAN is the most common NBIA accounting for roughly half of all cases [12]. In the 11 publications describing PKAN, all papers described patients with atypical features while three also described patients with typical Parkinsonism. The atypical features displayed in these patients were a poor levodopa response [13–16], a lack of asymmetrical features [15,17–19], or the presence of dystonia in addition to Parkinsonism [14,20–22] (Appendix B). In two publications, pyramidal signs were also observed [19,23]. Recent research has established that Lewy body pathology is not observed in PKAN, which may explain why atypical features of Parkinsonism are more commonly seen [24]. Historical reports of patients with PKAN have found α-synuclein inclusions in neurons [7,25]. However, Schneider et al. believe these patients may have been misdiagnosed since these reports were published before gene identification was available for diagnosing PKAN [24]. They describe a recent series of genetically confirmed PKAN patients in which all lacked any evidence of Lewy body pathology. This suggests a differing pathology is occurring in these patients. Our results showing a high prevalence of atypical Parkinsonism in PKAN sufferers supports this hypothesis. At the same time, the widespread presence of α-synuclein inclusions in the central nervous system (CNS) tissue of PLAN patients is well documented [26,27], which indicates a potential pathological link between PLAN and sporadic PD. The results from this review support this link with two of the three publications describing patients with PLAN due to features of typical Parkinsonism [28,29]. In the one paper describing atypical parkinsonism features in patients with PLAN, dystonia was present [30].

Hereditary haemochromatosis (HH) was also frequently identified in this systematic review. Four papers reported typical Parkinsonism [31–34] while atypical features were described in the remaining three papers. All papers were related to unresponsiveness to levodopa [35–37]. These reports of Parkinsonism and HH presenting concurrently indicate that research into iron accumulation in the CNS tissue of HH patients may clarify the pathological link between HH and PD.

The pathological processes and brain regions involved in HH are not well understood. In particular, the location of iron accumulation in CNS tissue is poorly documented. Since Parkinson's disease treatments were reported to be ineffective in these patients and an atypical picture was observed, it may be that a different area of the brain is affected. Further research is required in order to identify how and where the iron accumulation occurs in order to draw further conclusions from this result.

Six publications described Parkinsonism in Wilson's disease. It is well established that copper deposition, as seen in Wilson's disease patients, commonly has toxic effects in the brain, which leads to severe neurological features [38,39]. How copper causes neuronal death is not well understood even though it is generally accepted that the copper accumulates extracellularly and does not enter neurons [38]. Within this group, four publications described typical Parkinsonism in Wilson's disease [40–43] and two described atypical parkinsonism [44,45]. Although Parkinsonism is a common feature of neurologic Wilson's disease [38,39], there is no evidence to suggest that Wilson's disease causes Lewy body pathology. Despite this, all of the Wilson's Disease patients from this study displayed levodopa responsiveness. This included two patients with atypical parkinsonism where one had dystonia [44] and one had epilepsy [45]. As mitochondrial dysfunction plays a large role in the pathophysiology of PD [1,2], the extracellular accumulation of copper in the CNS may have the same effect on mitochondria within the neuron that it does within the hepatocytes. Despite the similarities in clinical features and the response to levodopa, these patients' demographics differ significantly to those seen in the sporadic PD population, which is outlined by Rizek et al. [46]. The average age of onset of Parkinsonism in these Wilson's disease patients was reported as 46 years old, which is considerably younger than in the sporadic PD population (mean age 65 years old). Furthermore, twice as many females as males were described as having Parkinsonism, which differs greatly to the ratio of 1.5 males per females seen in the sporadic PD population. However, since only nine patients were described, this is not a large enough population to draw generalizable conclusions especially since the lack of α-synuclein pathology indicates the presence of a different pathological process.

Despite previous research establishing that cigarette smoking is protective for PD [4], the smoking status was not reported in any of the publications (Appendix B). Therefore, it was not possible to investigate this in the current study. It would be pertinent to include the smoking status in the patient demographics of all future publications describing PD or features of Parkinsonism.

The precise nature of the relationship between iron accumulation in patients with Parkinsonism is not clear. Autopsy studies were excluded from this review since they offered retrospective details of the clinical picture and the timelines were poorly outlined. However, they could yield some useful findings in patients with metal storage disorders. Post mortem brain studies on patients with NBIAs allows us to investigate the correlation between the quantity of iron and the severity of PD features. Should this confirm that iron accumulation in the brain leads to the development of Parkinsonism, it follows that treatments to reduce the CNS iron levels, or act as an iron chelator, could be developed as an early treatment for patients with sporadic PD in order to delay the Parkinsonian features.

An important factor to consider when interpreting these results is the level and quality of evidence available in the literature. The majority of the publications included were case reports and case series that the Oxford Centre of Evidence-Based Medicine considers level 4 evidence [47]. However, due to the rarity of these individual IEMs, this was the highest level of evidence available. Case reports can be subject to bias and, although no formal bias assessment was conducted, a more favourable response to levodopa or exaggeration of the severity of the features may have been reported. This was taken into consideration when evaluating articles for inclusion and any paper describing a response less than moderate to levodopa was classed as atypical.

5. Conclusions

In conclusion, the presence of Parkinsonism in metal storage disorders is an under reported topic. Establishing the relationships between these conditions may clarify the pathological mechanisms of

Parkinsonism. Therefore, it is a field of growing interest with the number of publications describing patients with metal storage disorders displaying Parkinsonism growing substantially each decade. This review has demonstrated the following:

1. There is evidence of Parkinsonism coexisting with metal storage disorders in particular neurodegenerative brain iron accumulation disorders.
2. Patients with these metal storage disorders have an earlier age of onset of Parkinsonism than sporadic PD patients, which suggests additional underlying pathological processes are taking place. The ratio of males to females seen in many of these also differs significantly to the sporadic PD population, which further indicates a differing pathogenesis.
3. Future research must be conducted at a higher level than individual case reports to better assess the relationship between metal storage disorders and Parkinsonism. Cohort studies or case control studies using large cohorts will lead to a reliable dataset. At the same time, research in sporadic PD patients will identify whether any of the pathological mutations or processes are involved in the disorders discussed in relation to the development of Parkinsonism.
4. Smoking status and ethnicity should be documented in all future studies of Parkinsonism since Caucasian ethnicity is a large risk factor in sporadic PD while cigarette smoking appears to be protective. Recording these demographics will allow for the investigation of their presence in patients with metal storage disorders.

Author Contributions: E.B.: Main reviewer, developing, constructing, and proofing the article. Editing figures and corresponding author. J.G.: Second reviewer, constructing, proofing, and editing the article. E.E.B.: Senior reviewer, concept design, proofing, and editing the article.

Funding: This is a summary of independent research carried out at the National Institute for Health Research (NIHR) Sheffield Biomedical Research Centre (Translational Neuroscience). The views expressed are those of the author(s) and not necessarily those of the NHS, the NIHR, or the Department of Health.

Acknowledgments: The authors would like to thank Alisdair McNeill for the initial research concept, support during development of the review protocol, and his advice in the development of this manuscript.

Conflicts of Interest: The authors declare no conflict of interest.

Appendix A.

Search terms. Term A: Parkinson, Parkinson's, Parkinsonism, Parkinsonism. Term B: Aceruloplasminemia, Acrodermatitis, Bartter disease, BPAN, Calcium metabolism, CoPAN, Copper metabolism, DiGeorge, Fahr, Hemochromatosis, Hereditary rickets, Iron metabolism, Kufor-Rakeb syndrome, Magnesium metabolism, Menkes, Mitochondrial membrane protein-associated neurodegeneration, Neurodegenerative brain iron accumulation, Neuroferritinopathy, PLAN, PLA2G6-associated neurodegeneration, Phosphate metabolism, Pseudohypoparathyroidism, Tumoral calcinosis, Vitamin D metabolism, Wilson, Woodhouse-Sakati syndrome, Zinc metabolism.

Appendix B.

Table A1. Table showing the individual breakdown of the included publications. NA = Not Available.

Paper	Type of Paper	Condition	Male/Female	Average Age at Onset of Parkinsonism (years)	Ethnicity	Smoking Status	Typical Parkinsonism	Atypical Parkinsonism	Parkinsonism Features
Alberca, R. et al., 1987. [20]	Case report	PKAN	1M/1F	27	NA	NA	✓		Female siblings: Typical features. Male sibling; associated with dystonia. Fast progression.
Batla, A. et al., 015. [48]	Case report	Neuroferritinopathy	1F	79	NA	NA		✓	Associated with dystonia.
Behrens, M.I. et al., 2010. [49]	Case Series	Kufor-Rakeb Syndrome	4M/1F	NA	Chilean	NA		✓	Parkinsonian features in all five pts. No tremor present. Supranuclear gaze palsy in 4/5, poor L-dopa response
Bozi, M. et al., 2009. [23]	Case report	PKAN	1M	15	NA	NA		✓	Mildly affected but associated with pyramidal signs.
Chinnery, P.F. et al., 2007. [50]	Cross-sectional study	Neuroferritinopathy	3F	NA	2 English, 1 French	NA		✓	Associated with dystonia in all three. No tremor present.
Costello, D.J. et al., 2004. [31]	Case report	Hereditary Haemochromatosis	3M/1F	53	NA	NA	✓		Four pts all with HH and IPD diagnoses, classical signs. Good L-dopa response.
Crosiers, D. et al., 2011. [51]	case report	Kufor-Rakeb syndrome	1M	10	Afghan	NA		✓	Associated with dystonia.
Czlonkowska, A. et al., 2018. [40]	Cross-sectional study	Wilson's disease	NA	NA	Polish	NA	✓		Parkinsonism found in 11.3% (6/53 pts).
Darling, A. et al., 2017. [21]	Cross-sectional study	PKAN	22M/25F	NA	NA	NA		✓	Features of Parkinsonism displayed in all 47 pts. Associated with Dystonia. Bradykinesia and rigidity on left side. Poor L-dopa response.
Demarquay, G. et al., 2000. [35]	Case report	Hereditary Haemochromatosis	2M/1F	56	NA	NA		✓	Features of Parkinsonism in all three pts. Supranuclear gaze palsy and hallucinations/ psychotic episodes in 1/3, psychotic episodes in 1/3, and typical features in 1/3.
Di Fonzo, A. et al., 2007. [52]	Cross-sectional study	Kufor-Rakeb Syndrome	3M	NA	NA	NA	✓		L-dopa unresponsive, symmetrical features.
Diaz, N., 2013. [13]	Case report	PKAN	1F	NA	NA	NA		✓	Supranuclear gaze palsy, cognitive impairment, and hallucinations.
Eiberg, H. et al., 2012. [53]	Case report	Kufor-Rakeb Syndrome	1M	12	NA	NA		✓	Rest tremor and bradykinesia with mental retardation.
Evans, B.K. & Donley, D.K., 1988. [54]	Case report	Pseudohypoparathyroidism	1F	20	NA	NA		✓	Typical features. Poor L-dopa response but dystonia present upon removal of L-dopa.
Fekete, R., 2012. [55]	Case report	NBIA, unknown type	1M	73	NA	NA	✓		Mild typical parkinsonism.
Fonderico, M. et al., 2017. [56]	Case report	BPAN	1F	26	NA	NA			
Gasca-Salas, C. et al., 2017. [44]	Case report	Wilson's Disease	1F	38	NA	NA		✓	Tremor, clumsiness, rigidity, and dystonia in left arm. Good L-dopa response.

Table A1. Cont.

Paper	Type of Paper	Condition	Male/Female	Average Age at Onset of Parkinsonism (years)	Ethnicity	Smoking Status	Typical Parkinsonism	Atypical Parkinsonism	Parkinsonism Features
Giri, A. et al., 2016. [28]	Case report	PLAN	1F	27	NA	NA	✓		Typical Features, PD diagnosis.
Girotra, T., Mahajan, A. & Sidiropoulos, C., 2017. [32]	Case report	Hereditary Haemochromatosis	1M	41	Caucasian	NA	✓		Typical features, mild but clear response to L-dopa.
Gondim, F. de A.A. et al., 2014. [41]	Case Series	Wilson's disease	2M/2F	28	Brazil	NA	✓		Four pts with typical features, all responded well to L-dopa.
Gore, E. et al., 2016. [57]	Case report	MPAN	1M	35	Kuwaiti	NA		✓	Developmental delay, dystonia, and parkinsonism. L-dopa responsive.
Hayflick, SJ. et al., 2013. [58]	Cohort study	BPAN	3M/18F	25	NA	NA		✓	Supranuclear gaze palsy, dystonia, and no L-dopa response.
Hermann, A. et al., 2017. [59]	Case report	BPAN	1F	24	German	NA		✓	Associated with dystonia
Ichinose, Y. et al., 2014. [60]	Case report	BPAN	1F	30	NA	NA		✓	Associated with dystonia in 2/2 pts.
Kim, YJ. et al., 2015. [30]	Case Series	PLAN	1M/1F	14	Korean	NA		✓	Chorea, dystonia, and psychological manifestations.
Klysz, B., Skowronska, M. & Kmiec, T., 2014. [61]	Case report	MPAN	1F	15	NA	NA		✓	Parkinsonian signs in three pts. One responded well to L-dopa, one not treated.
Kumar, N. et al., 2016. [33]	Case Series	Hereditary Haemochromatosis	2M/1F	59	1 Irish-Portuguese, 1 Scottish, 1 unknown	NA	✓		Typical parkinsonism in one pt though onset at 18. Bilateral features in the other.
Lee, C.-H. et al., 2013. [17]	Case report	PKAN	2M	20	Taiwanese	NA		✓	Poor response to L-dopa in all.
Lee, J.-H. et al., 2016. [14]	Cross-sectional study	PKAN	6M	36	NA	NA	✓		Associated with dystonia in 4/6 pts, isolated parkinsonism in 2/6 pts.
Mak, C.M. et al., 2011. [18]	Case report	PKAN	1M	27	Hong Kong	NA		✓	Bilateral features.
Ni, W. et al., 2016. [62]	Case report	Neuroferritinopathy	1F	44	NA	NA		✓	No response to L-dopa, pyramidal signs.
Nielsen, J.E., Jensen, L.N. & Krabbe, K., 1995. [34]	Case report	Hereditary Haemochromatosis	1M	29	NA	NA	✓		Typical PD features, immediate improvement with L-dopa.
Nishioka, K. et al., 2015. [63]	Cross-sectional study	BPAN	7F	32	NA	NA		✓	Cognitive dysfunction as presenting symptom in all seven. Otherwise typical parkinsonism. L-dopa responsive.
Oder, W. et al., 1991. [42]	Cross-sectional study	Wilson's Disease	NA	NA	NA	NA	✓		8/25 pts with parkinsonian features. Bradykinesia, resting tremor present. 9/15 pts with parkinsonian features.
Olgiati, S. et al., 2017. [64]	Cross-sectional study	MPAN	NA	NA	NA	NA		✓	Cognitive impairment and pyramidal signs seen.
Pearson, D.W. et al., 1981. [65]	Case report	Pseudohypoparathyroidism	1M	58	NA	NA		✓	Typical PD features. Very fast disease progression.
Pestana Knight, E.M., Gilman, S. & Selwa, L., 2009. [45]	Case report	Wilson's Disease	1M	55	NA	NA		✓	Typical PD features associated with epilepsy.

Table A1. Cont.

Paper	Type of Paper	Condition	Male/Female	Average Age at Onset of Parkinsonism (years)	Ethnicity	Smoking Status	Typical Parkinsonism	Atypical Parkinsonism	Parkinsonism Features
Racette, B.A. et al., 2001. [15]	Case report	PKAN	1F	60	NA	NA		✓	Bilateral features, no response to L-dopa.
Rohani, M. et al., 2017. [66]	Case report	Fahr disease	1F	50	NA	NA	✓		Typical L-dopa responsive parkinsonism.
Rosana, A. & La Rosa, L., 2007. [36]	Case report	Hereditary Haemochromatosis	1M	58	NA	NA		✓	No response to L-dopa.
Sakarya, A., Oncu, B. & Elibol, B., 2012. [19]	Case report	PKAN	1M	16	NA	NA		✓	Early severe cognitive impairment, bilateral onset, pyramidal features.
Scale, T. et al., 2014. [67]	Case report	Fahr Disease	1M	62	NA	NA		✓	No response to L-dopa.
Schneider, S.A. et al., 2010. [12]	Case report	Kufor-Rakeb syndrome	1M	16	Pakistan	NA		✓	Associated with dystonia.
Sechi, G. et al., 2007. [43]	Case report	Wilson's disease	3F	70	NA	NA	✓		Very late onset L-dopa responsive parkinsonism.
Seo, J.-H., Song, S.-K. & Lee, P.H., 2009. [16]	Case report	PKAN	1M	35	NA	NA		✓	No response to L-dopa.
Song, C.-Y. et al., 2017. [68]	Case report	Pseudohypoparathyroidism	1F	52	NA	NA		✓	Very fast disease progression.
Thomas, M., Hayflick, S.J. & Jankovic, J., 2004. [22]	Cross-sectional study	PKAN	14M/8F	35	NA	NA	✓		Typical parkinsonism seen, though clinical features not defined. Associated with dystonia in 4/22 pts.
Vroegindeweij, L.H.P. et al., 2017. [69]	Case Series	Aceruloplasminemia	4M/1F	NA	4 Dutch, 1 Italian	NA			Parkinsonian features in all pts. Associated with cognitive decline and cerebellar features in all pts.
Williams, S. et al., 2013. [37]	Case report	Hereditary Haemochromatosis	1F	60	Caucasian	NA		✓	Short disease course, early autonomic involvement, no L-dopa response.
Xie, F. et al., 2015. [29]	Case report	PLAN	2M	34	NA	NA	✓		Typical features, good L-dopa response.

References

1. Lubbe, S.; Morris, H.R. Recent advances in Parkinson's disease genetics. *J. Neurol.* **2014**, *261*, 259–266. [CrossRef] [PubMed]
2. Kalia, L.V.; Lang, A.E. Parkinson's disease. *Lancet (Lond. Engl.)* **2015**, *386*, 896–912. [CrossRef]
3. Noyce, A.J.; Bestwick, J.P.; Silveira-Moriyama, L.; Hawkes, C.H.; Giovannoni, G.; Lees, A.J.; Schrag, A. Meta-analysis of early nonmotor features and risk factors for Parkinson disease. *Ann. Neurol.* **2012**, *72*, 893–901. [CrossRef] [PubMed]
4. Kieburtz, K.; Wunderle, K.B. Parkinson's disease: Evidence for environmental risk factors. *Mov. Disord.* **2013**, *28*, 8–13. [CrossRef] [PubMed]
5. Deutschlander, A.B.; Ross, O.A.; Dickson, D.W.; Wszolek, Z.K. Atypical parkinsonian syndromes: A general neurologist's perspective. *Eur. J. Neurol.* **2018**, *25*, 41–58. [CrossRef] [PubMed]
6. Sanderson, S.; Green, A.; Preece, M.A.; Burton, H. The incidence of inherited metabolic disorders in the West Midlands, UK. *Arch. Dis. Child.* **2006**, *91*, 896–899. [CrossRef] [PubMed]
7. Waber, L. Inborn errors of metabolism. *Pediatr. Ann.* **1990**, *19*, 105–118. [CrossRef] [PubMed]
8. Pietracupa, S.; Martin-Bastida, A.; Piccini, P. Iron metabolism and its detection through MRI in parkinsonian disorders: A systematic review. *Neurol. Sci. Off. J. Ital. Neurol. Soc. Ital. Soc. Clin. Neurophysiol.* **2017**, *38*, 2095–2101. [CrossRef] [PubMed]
9. Mochizuki, H.; Yasuda, T. Iron accumulation in Parkinson's disease. *J. Neural Transm.* **2012**, *119*, 1511–1514. [CrossRef] [PubMed]
10. Moher, D.; Liberati, A.; Tetzlaff, J.; Altman, D.G.; Group, T.P. Preferred Reporting Items for Systematic Reviews and Meta-Analyses: The PRISMA Statement. *PLOS Med.* **2009**, *6*, e1000097. [CrossRef] [PubMed]
11. Ferreira, C.R.; Gahl, W.A. Disorders of metal metabolism. *Transl. Sci. Rare Dis.* **2017**, *2*, 101–139. [CrossRef] [PubMed]
12. Schneider, S.; Paisan-Ruiz, C.; Quinn, N.; Lees, A.; MD, F.; Houlden, H.; Hardy, J.; Bhatia, K.P. ATP13A2 mutations (PARK9) cause neurodegeneration with brain iron accumulation. *Mov. Disord.* **2010**, *25*, 979–984. [CrossRef] [PubMed]
13. Diaz, N. Late onset atypical pantothenate-kinase-associated neurodegeneration. *Case Rep. Neurol. Med.* **2013**, *2013*, 860201. [CrossRef] [PubMed]
14. Lee, J.-H.; Park, J.; Ryu, H.-S.; Park, H.; Kim, Y.E.; Hong, J.Y.; Nam, S.O.; Sung, Y.-H.; Lee, S.-H.; Lee, J.-Y.; et al. Clinical Heterogeneity of Atypical Pantothenate Kinase-Associated Neurodegeneration in Koreans. *J. Mov. Disord.* **2016**, *9*, 20–27. [CrossRef] [PubMed]
15. Racette, B.A.; Perry, A.; D'Avossa, G.; Perlmutter, J.S. Late-onset neurodegeneration with brain iron accumulation type 1: Expanding the clinical spectrum. *Mov. Disord.* **2001**, *16*, 1148–1152. [CrossRef] [PubMed]
16. Seo, J.-H.; Song, S.-K.; Lee, P.H. A Novel PANK2 Mutation in a Patient with Atypical Pantothenate-Kinase-Associated Neurodegeneration Presenting with Adult-Onset Parkinsonism. *J. Clin. Neurol.* **2009**, *5*, 192–194. [CrossRef] [PubMed]
17. Lee, C.-H.; Lu, C.-S.; Chuang, W.-L.; Yeh, T.-H.; Jung, S.-M.; Huang, C.-L.; Lai, S.-C. Phenotypes and genotypes of patients with pantothenate kinase-associated neurodegeneration in Asian and Caucasian populations: 2 cases and literature review. *Sci. World J.* **2013**, *2013*, 860539. [CrossRef] [PubMed]
18. Mak, C.M.; Sheng, B.; Lee, H.H.; Lau, K.; Chan, W.; Lam, C.; Chan, Y. Young-onset parkinsonism in a Hong Kong Chinese man with adult-onset Hallervorden-Spatz syndrome. *Int. J. Neurosci.* **2011**, *121*, 224–227. [CrossRef] [PubMed]
19. Sakarya, A.; Oncu, B.; Elibol, B. Panthothenate kinase-associated neurodegeneration (PKAN) presenting with language deterioration, personality alteration, and severe parkinsonism. *J. Neuropsychiatry Clin. Neurosci.* **2012**, *24*, E13–E14. [CrossRef] [PubMed]
20. Alberca, R.; Rafel, E.; Chinchon, I.; Vadillo, J.; Navarro, A. Late onset parkinsonian syndrome in Hallervorden-Spatz disease. *J. Neurol. Neurosurg. Psychiatry* **1987**, *50*, 1665–1668. [CrossRef] [PubMed]
21. Darling, A.; Tello, C.; Marti, M.J.; Garrido, C.; Aguilera-Albesa, S.; Tomas Vila, M.; Gaston, I.; Madruga, M.; Gonzalez Gutierrez, L.; Ramos Lizana, J.; et al. Clinical rating scale for pantothenate kinase-associated neurodegeneration: A pilot study. *Mov. Disord.* **2017**, *32*, 1620–1630. [CrossRef] [PubMed]

22. Thomas, M.; Hayflick, S.J.; Jankovic, J. Clinical heterogeneity of neurodegeneration with brain iron accumulation (Hallervorden-Spatz syndrome) and pantothenate kinase-associated neurodegeneration. *Mov. Disord.* **2004**, *19*, 36–42. [CrossRef] [PubMed]
23. Bozi, M.; Matarin, M.; Theocharis, I.; Potagas, C.; Stefanis, L. A patient with pantothenate kinase-associated neurodegeneration and supranuclear gaze palsy. *Clin. Neurol. Neurosurg.* **2009**, *111*, 688–690. [CrossRef] [PubMed]
24. Schneider, S.A.; Dusek, P.; Hardy, J.; Westenberger, A.; Jankovic, J.; Bhatia, K.P. Genetics and Pathophysiology of Neurodegeneration with Brain Iron Accumulation (NBIA). *Curr. Neuropharmacol.* **2013**, *11*, 59–79. [CrossRef] [PubMed]
25. Saito, Y.; Kawai, M.; Inoue, K.; Sasaki, R.; Arai, H.; Nanba, E.; Kuzuhara, S.; Ihara, Y.; Kanazawa, I.; Murayama, S. Widespread expression of alpha-synuclein and tau immunoreactivity in Hallervorden-Spatz syndrome with protracted clinical course. *J. Neurol. Sci.* **2000**, *177*, 48–59. [CrossRef]
26. Gregory, A.; Westaway, S.K.; Holm, I.E.; Kotzbauer, P.T.; Hogarth, P.; Sonek, S.; Coryell, J.C.; Nguyen, T.M.; Nardocci, N.; Zorzi, G.; et al. Neurodegeneration associated with genetic defects in phospholipase A(2). *Neurology* **2008**, *71*, 1402–1409. [CrossRef] [PubMed]
27. Paisan-Ruiz, C.; Li, A.; Schneider, S.A.; Holton, J.L.; Johnson, R.; Kidd, D.; Chataway, J.; Bhatia, K.P.; Lees, A.J.; Hardy, J.; et al. Widespread Lewy body and tau accumulation in childhood and adult onset dystonia-parkinsonism cases with PLA2G6 mutations. *Neurobiol. Aging* **2012**, *33*, 814–823. [CrossRef] [PubMed]
28. Giri, A.; Guven, G.; Hanagasi, H.; Hauser, A.-K.; Erginul-Unaltuna, N.; Bilgic, B.; Gurvit, H.; Heutink, P.; Gasser, T.; Lohmann, E.; et al. PLA2G6 Mutations Related to Distinct Phenotypes: A New Case with Early-onset Parkinsonism. *Tremor Other Hyperkinet. Mov. (N. Y.)* **2016**, *6*, 363. [CrossRef]
29. Xie, F.; Cen, Z.; Ouyang, Z.; Wu, S.; Xiao, J.; Luo, W. Homozygous p.D331Y mutation in PLA2G6 in two patients with pure autosomal-recessive early-onset parkinsonism: further evidence of a fourth phenotype of PLA2G6-associated neurodegeneration. *Parkinsonism Relat. Disord.* **2015**, *21*, 420–422. [CrossRef] [PubMed]
30. Kim, Y.J.; Lyoo, C.H.; Hong, S.; Kim, N.Y.; Lee, M.S. Neuroimaging studies and whole exome sequencing of PLA2G6-associated neurodegeneration in a family with intrafamilial phenotypic heterogeneity. *Parkinsonism Relat. Disord.* **2015**, *21*, 402–406. [CrossRef] [PubMed]
31. Costello, D.J.; Walsh, S.L.; Harrington, H.J.; Walsh, C.H. Concurrent hereditary haemochromatosis and idiopathic Parkinson's disease: A case report series. *J. Neurol. Neurosurg. Psychiatry* **2004**, *75*, 631–633. [CrossRef] [PubMed]
32. Girotra, T.; Mahajan, A.; Sidiropoulos, C. Levodopa Responsive Parkinsonism in Patients with Hemochromatosis: Case Presentation and Literature Review. *Case Rep. Neurol. Med.* **2017**, *2017*, 5146723. [CrossRef] [PubMed]
33. Kumar, N.; Rizek, P.; Sadikovic, B.; Adams, P.C.; Jog, M. Movement Disorders Associated With Hemochromatosis. *Can. J. Neurol. Sci.* **2016**, *43*, 801–808. [CrossRef] [PubMed]
34. Nielsen, J.E.; Jensen, L.N.; Krabbe, K. Hereditary haemochromatosis: A case of iron accumulation in the basal ganglia associated with a parkinsonian syndrome. *J. Neurol. Neurosurg. Psychiatry* **1995**, *59*, 318–321. [CrossRef] [PubMed]
35. Demarquay, G.; Setiey, A.; Morel, Y.; Trepo, C.; Chazot, G.; Broussolle, E. Clinical report of three patients with hereditary hemochromatosis and movement disorders. *Mov. Disord.* **2000**, *15*, 1204–1209. [CrossRef]
36. Rosana, A.; La Rosa, L. A case of hereditary haemochromatosis in a patient with extrapyramidal syndrome. *Blood Transfus.* **2007**, *5*, 241–243. [CrossRef] [PubMed]
37. Williams, S.; Vinjam, M.R.; Ismail, A.; Hassan, A. A parkinsonian movement disorder with brain iron deposition and a haemochromatosis mutation. *J. Neurol.* **2013**, *260*, 2170–2171. [CrossRef] [PubMed]
38. Ferenci, P. Pathophysiology and clinical features of Wilson disease. *Metab. Brain Dis.* **2004**, *19*, 229–239. [CrossRef] [PubMed]
39. Lorincz, M.T. Neurologic Wilson's disease. *Ann. N. Y. Acad. Sci.* **2010**, *1184*, 173–187. [CrossRef] [PubMed]
40. Czlonkowska, A.; Litwin, T.; Dziezyc, K.; Karlinski, M.; Bring, J.; Bjartmar, C. Characteristics of a newly diagnosed Polish cohort of patients with neurological manifestations of Wilson disease evaluated with the Unified Wilson's Disease Rating Scale. *BMC Neurol.* **2018**, *18*, 34. [CrossRef] [PubMed]
41. De Gondim, F.A.; Araujo, D.F.; Oliveira, I.S.; Vale, O.C. Small fiber dysfunction in patients with Wilson's disease. *Arq. Neuropsiquiatr.* **2014**, *72*, 592–595. [CrossRef]

42. Oder, W.; Grimm, G.; Kollegger, H.; Ferenci, P.; Schneider, B.; Deecke, L. Neurological and neuropsychiatric spectrum of Wilson's disease: A prospective study of 45 cases. *J. Neurol.* **1991**, *238*, 281–287. [PubMed]
43. Sechi, G.; Antonio Cocco, G.; Errigo, A.; Deiana, L.; Rosati, G.; Agnetti, V.; Stephen Paulus, K.; Mario Pes, G. Three sisters with very-late-onset major depression and parkinsonism. *Parkinsonism Relat. Disord.* **2007**, *13*, 122–125. [CrossRef] [PubMed]
44. Gasca-Salas, C.; Alonso, A.; Gonzalez-Redondo, R.; Obeso, J.A. Coexisting Parkinson's and Wilson's Disease: Chance or Connection? *Can. J. Neurol. Sci.* **2017**, *44*, 215–218. [CrossRef] [PubMed]
45. Pestana Knight, E.M.; Gilman, S.; Selwa, L. Status epilepticus in Wilson's disease. *Epileptic Disord.* **2009**, *11*, 138–143. [CrossRef] [PubMed]
46. Rizek, P.; Kumar, N.; Jog, M.S. An update on the diagnosis and treatment of Parkinson disease. *Can. Med. Assoc. J.* **2016**, *188*, 1157–1165. [CrossRef] [PubMed]
47. Oxford Centre for Evidence-Based Medicine—Levels of Evidence (March 2009). 2009. Available online: https://www.cebm.net/2009/06/oxford-centre-evidence-based-medicine-levels-evidence-march-2009/ (accessed on 29 July 2018).
48. Batla, A.; Adams, M.E.; Erro, R.; Ganos, C.; Balint, B.; Mencacci, N.E.; Bhatia, K.P. Cortical pencil lining in neuroferritinopathy: A diagnostic clue. *Neurology* **2015**, *84*, 1816–1818. [CrossRef] [PubMed]
49. Behrens, M.I.; Bruggemann, N.; Chana, P.; Venegas, P.; Kagi, M.; Parrao, T.; Orellana, P.; Garrido, C.; Rojas, C.V.; Hauke, J.; et al. Clinical spectrum of Kufor-Rakeb syndrome in the Chilean kindred with ATP13A2 mutations. *Mov. Disord.* **2010**, *25*, 1929–1937. [CrossRef] [PubMed]
50. Chinnery, P.F.; Crompton, D.E.; Birchall, D.; Jackson, M.J.; Coulthard, A.; Lombes, A.; Quinn, N.; Wills, A.; Fletcher, N.; Mottershead, J.P.; et al. Clinical features and natural history of neuroferritinopathy caused by the FTL1 460InsA mutation. *Brain* **2007**, *130*, 110–119. [CrossRef] [PubMed]
51. Crosiers, D.; Ceulemans, B.; Meeus, B.; Nuytemans, K.; Pals, P.; van Broeckhoven, C.; Cras, P.; Theuns, J. Juvenile dystonia-parkinsonism and dementia caused by a novel ATP13A2 frameshift mutation. *Parkinsonism Relat. Disord.* **2011**, *17*, 135–138. [CrossRef] [PubMed]
52. Di Fonzo, A.; Chien, H.F.; Socal, M.; Giraudo, S.; Tassorelli, C.; Iliceto, G.; Fabbrini, G.; Marconi, R.; Fincati, E.; Abbruzzese, G.; et al. ATP13A2 missense mutations in juvenile parkinsonism and young onset Parkinson disease. *Neurology* **2007**, *68*, 1557–1562. [CrossRef] [PubMed]
53. Eiberg, H.; Hansen, L.; Korbo, L.; Nielsen, I.M.; Svenstrup, K.; Bech, S.; Pinborg, L.H.; Friberg, L.; Hjermind, L.E.; Olsen, O.R.; et al. Novel mutation in ATP13A2 widens the spectrum of Kufor-Rakeb syndrome (PARK9). *Clin. Genet.* **2012**, *82*, 256–263. [CrossRef] [PubMed]
54. Evans, B.K.; Donley, D.K. Pseudohypoparathyroidism, parkinsonism syndrome, with no basal ganglia calcification. *J. Neurol. Neurosurg. Psychiatry* **1988**, *51*, 709–713. [CrossRef] [PubMed]
55. Fekete, R. Late onset neurodegeneration with brain-iron accumulation presenting as parkinsonism. *Case Rep. Neurol. Med.* **2012**, *2012*, 387095. [CrossRef] [PubMed]
56. Fonderico, M.; Laudisi, M.; Andreasi, N.G.; Bigoni, S.; Lamperti, C.; Panteghini, C.; Garavaglia, B.; Carecchio, M.; Emanuele, E.A.; Gian, L.F.; et al. Patient Affected by Beta-Propeller Protein-Associated Neurodegeneration: A Therapeutic Attempt with Iron Chelation Therapy. *Front. Neurol.* **2017**, *8*, 385. [CrossRef] [PubMed]
57. Gore, E.; Appleby, B.S.; Cohen, M.L.; DeBrosse, S.D.; Leverenz, J.B.; Miller, B.L.; Siedlak, S.L.; Zhu, X.; Lerner, A.J. Clinical and imaging characteristics of late onset mitochondrial membrane protein-associated neurodegeneration (MPAN). *Neurocase* **2016**, *22*, 476–483. [CrossRef] [PubMed]
58. Hayflick, S.J.; Kruer, M.C.; Gregory, A.; Haack, T.B.; Kurian, M.A.; Houlden, H.H.; Anderson, J.; Boddaert, N.; Sanford, L.; Harik, S.I.; et al. Beta-Propeller protein-associated neurodegeneration: A new X-linked dominant disorder with brain iron accumulation. *Brain* **2013**, *136*, 1708–1717. [CrossRef] [PubMed]
59. Hermann, A.; Kitzler, H.H.; Pollack, T.; Biskup, S.; Kruger, S.; Funke, C.; Terrile, C.; Haack, T.B. A Case of Beta-propeller Protein-associated Neurodegeneration due to a Heterozygous Deletion of WDR45. *Tremor Other Hyperkinet. Mov. (N. Y.)* **2017**, *7*, 465. [CrossRef]
60. Ichinose, Y.; Miwa, M.; Onohara, A.; Obi, K.; Shindo, K.; Saitsu, H.; Matsumoto, N.; Takiyama, Y. Characteristic MRI findings in beta-propeller protein-associated neurodegeneration (BPAN). *Neurol. Clin. Pract.* **2014**, *4*, 175–177. [CrossRef] [PubMed]
61. Klysz, B.; Skowronska, M.; Kmiec, T. Mitochondrial protein associated neurodegeneration—Case report. *Neurol. Neurochir. Pol.* **2014**, *48*, 81–84. [CrossRef] [PubMed]

62. Ni, W.; Li, H.-F.; Zheng, Y.-C.; Wu, Z.-Y. FTL mutation in a Chinese pedigree with neuroferritinopathy. *Neurol. Genet.* **2016**, *2*, e74. [CrossRef] [PubMed]
63. Nishioka, K.; Oyama, G.; Yoshino, H.; Li, Y.; Matsushima, T.; Takeuchi, C.; Mochizuki, Y.; Mori-Yoshimura, M.; Murata, M.; Yamasita, C.; et al. High frequency of beta-propeller protein-associated neurodegeneration (BPAN) among patients with intellectual disability and young-onset parkinsonism. *Neurobiol. Aging* **2015**, *36*, 2004.e9–2004.e15. [CrossRef] [PubMed]
64. Olgiati, S.; Dogu, O.; Tufekcioglu, Z.; Diler, Y.; Saka, E.; Gultekin, M.; Kaleagasi, H.; Kuipers, D.; Graafland, J.; Breedveld, G.J.; et al. The p.Thr11Met mutation in c19orf12 is frequent among adult Turkish patients with MPAN. *Parkinsonism Relat. Disord.* **2017**, *39*, 64–70. [CrossRef] [PubMed]
65. Pearson, D.W.; Durward, W.F.; Fogelman, I.; Boyle, I.T.; Beastall, G. Pseudohypoparathyroidism presenting as severe Parkinsonism. *Postgrad. Med. J.* **1981**, *57*, 445–447. [CrossRef] [PubMed]
66. Rohani, M.; Poon, Y.-Y.; Naranian, T.; Fasano, A. SCL20A2 mutation mimicking fluctuating Parkinson's disease. *Parkinsonism Relat. Disord.* **2017**, *39*, 93–94. [CrossRef] [PubMed]
67. Scale, T.; Lewis, C.; Hedayat, A.; Bilal, M.; Wani, M. Cerebral calcification from Fahr's disease with co-existing haemochromatosis. *Prog. Neurol. Psychiatry* **2014**, *18*, 14–16. [CrossRef]
68. Song, C.-Y.; Zhao, Z.-X.; Li, W.; Sun, C.-C.; Liu, Y.-M. Pseudohypoparathyroidism with basal ganglia calcification: A case report of rare cause of reversible parkinsonism. *Medicine (Baltim.)* **2017**, *96*, e6312. [CrossRef] [PubMed]
69. Vroegindeweij, L.H.P.; Langendonk, J.G.; Langeveld, M.; Hoogendoorn, M.; Kievit, A.J.A.; Di Raimondo, D.; Wilson, J.H.P.; Boon, A.J.W. New insights in the neurological phenotype of aceruloplasminemia in Caucasian patients. *Parkinsonism Relat. Disord.* **2017**, *36*, 33–40. [CrossRef] [PubMed]

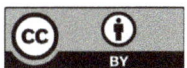 © 2018 by the authors. Licensee MDPI, Basel, Switzerland. This article is an open access article distributed under the terms and conditions of the Creative Commons Attribution (CC BY) license (http://creativecommons.org/licenses/by/4.0/).

MDPI
St. Alban-Anlage 66
4052 Basel
Switzerland
Tel. +41 61 683 77 34
Fax +41 61 302 89 18
www.mdpi.com

Brain Sciences Editorial Office
E-mail: brainsci@mdpi.com
www.mdpi.com/journal/brainsci

www.ingramcontent.com/pod-product-compliance
Lightning Source LLC
LaVergne TN
LVHW072000080526
838202LV00064B/6803